THE HEALTHY HEART BLUEPRINT

A Comprehensive Plan to Transform Your Cardiovascular Well-Being Through Balanced Nutrition, Regular Exercise, Stress Reduction, & Restful Sleep for a Healthier Life

DR. JITESH ARORA

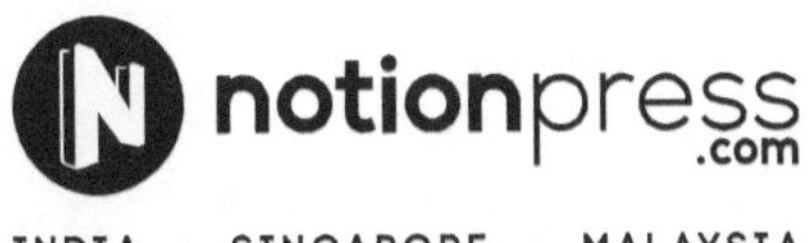

INDIA · SINGAPORE · MALAYSIA

Contents

Introduction

Embarking on Your Healthiest Heart Journey

Your heart beats more than 100,000 times each day – an awe-inspiring reminder of its tireless commitment to keeping you alive and well. Yet, amid the rapid pace of modern life, it is easy to forget how much care this remarkable organ truly deserves. What if, by making just a few thoughtful changes, you could protect your heart and transform your entire well-being?

In an era where convenience often takes precedence over health, focusing on heart care has never been more important. *Healthy Heart Blueprint* is your invitation to discover how small, purposeful steps can have a life-changing impact.

Who This Book Is For

Whether you are a parent striving to instil healthy habits in your family, a young adult eager to lay the groundwork for lifelong wellness, or a healthcare provider guiding others toward prevention, this book speaks to anyone who wants a clear path to a more vibrant, fulfilling life. If your goal is to safeguard your cardiovascular health—and by extension, your overall well-being — then *Healthy Heart Blueprint* is for you.

Why Heart Health Matters

Consider Maya, a busy working mother juggling career responsibilities, family obligations, and the daily pressures of a fast-paced world. A routine cholesterol test served as her wakeup call—she realised that change was not just an option but a necessity. One year later, her radiant energy and renewed confidence astonished everyone around her.

Maya's transformation was not magical; it resulted from replacing unhealthy habits with small, meaningful changes in her everyday routine. Her story is not out of the ordinary—and that is what makes it so empowering.

Like Maya, you have the power to nurture your heart through balanced nutrition, regular movement, restorative sleep, and supportive relationships. In the chapters ahead, you will learn how these choices can be both accessible and sustainable, helping you unlock your heart's full potential.

A Holistic Approach to Heart Health

True heart health goes beyond physical fitness. It encompasses your mental clarity, emotional resilience, and the quality of your relationships. In *Healthy Heart Blueprint*, you will explore how every aspect of your life—what you eat, how you move, how you rest, and how you connect with others—affects the strength and vitality of your cardiovascular system.

Imagine waking up each morning feeling refreshed, your mind and body aligned. Picture sitting down to meals that both delight your taste buds and support your health and engaging in activities that elevate your mood while fortifying your heart. This holistic vision is well within reach, and this book will guide you towards making the everyday choices that lead to a healthier heart and a more fulfilling life.

The Blueprint: Your Path to Lifelong Wellness

Healthy Heart Blueprint is more than just a set of guidelines – it is a supportive roadmap crafted for a diverse range of readers:

- **Families:** Build health-focused traditions that bring everyone closer. Turn shared meals and activities into long-term habits that enrich each generation.

- **Young Adults:** Form healthy choices early so they become second nature, laying the groundwork for lasting wellness.

- **Healthcare Providers:** Discover practical, evidence-based strategies to inspire and empower patients with meaningful heart care.

Through relatable stories, the latest research, and clear, actionable advice, this book demystifies heart health, proving it is achievable regardless of your starting point.

What You'll Discover

1. Heart-Friendly Nutrition

Enjoy meals that satisfy your cravings while nourishing your body. Uncover recipes and ingredients that make eating well feel like a gratifying act of self-care.

2. Movement That Inspires

From brisk walks to joyful dance sessions, find exercises that fit seamlessly into your schedule and turn staying active into a source of daily enjoyment.

3. Stress Resilience

Learn mindfulness practices and stress management techniques to stay centred. Protect your heart by cultivating calm and clarity in both mind and body.

4. Restorative Sleep

Discover the profound impact of quality sleep on your heart and overall vitality. Explore strategies that help you create an environment conducive to deep, revitalising rest.

5. The Power of Connection

Strengthen relationships that bolster emotional well-being and support a resilient heart. See how meaningful social ties can become a central pillar of heart health.

Your Journey Begins Here

Healthy Heart Blueprint is your partner in an empowering journey. Through compassionate guidance, personal stories, and practical tips, you will gain the knowledge and motivation to take control of your cardiovascular well-being—one step at a time.

As you move through each chapter, you will collect valuable tools that help you build habits aligned with your goals and values. Every section builds on the one before it, creating a balanced lifestyle that enhances not just your physical health, but also your emotional and mental vitality.

This is your invitation to give yourself and your loved ones the gift of a stronger, happier heart. Let *Healthy Heart Blueprint* be your trusted companion, lighting the way towards a life defined by robust energy, peace of mind, and confidence that comes from genuinely caring for your heart.

Welcome to the beginning of a remarkable journey towards lifelong vitality. Your healthiest heart awaits.

Eat Smart for a Healthy Heart

Your heart is one of the most extraordinary organs in your body, beating over 100,000 times a day to sustain your life. Yet, it often goes unnoticed or underappreciated amid day-to-day stresses, deadlines, errands, and to do lists. We frequently take it for granted, trusting it to keep pumping tirelessly no matter how we treat our bodies. The truth is, however, that **nutrition**, the simple, daily act of eating—has a profound impact on how well your heart functions. The foods you choose, the way you prepare them, and how often you consume them can dramatically influence your energy levels, your sense of well-being, and your lifespan.

In many ways, food can be your greatest ally. By emphasising **evidence-based dietary principles**, you can transform your heart's health and support your entire cardiovascular system. Whether you are looking to reduce cholesterol, manage blood pressure, shed unwanted pounds, or simply live with more energy and vitality, your journey starts here. Each decision you make about what lands on your plate can become part of a powerful strategy to protect your heart—and support the ones you love.

Expanding Your Perspective on Heart Health

The biggest challenge for many of us is shifting our view of heart health from an abstract concept to a tangible, day-to-day reality. It is easy to look at a plate of food and see only calories, flavours, or convenience. But by **reframing how we perceive each meal**, we can cultivate a deeper understanding of how every ingredient either benefits or burdens our hearts. This shift allows us to see food as more than mere sustenance—food can be medicine, nourishment, and even a source of joy.

Equally important is recognising that heart health is a **collective effort**. Our dietary choices affect not only ourselves but also our families, communities, and even the healthcare system at large. When families commit to healthy eating, the results can be life-changing: improved quality of life, fewer doctor visits, more confidence, and a shared sense of unity around a common goal. Meanwhile, young adults who establish robust eating habits early can set the stage for decades of vitality and resilience.

In the following sections, you will learn about the **key pillars** of a heart-healthy diet. We'll explore nutrient-dense foods and their antioxidant properties, the intricacies of different types of fats and cholesterol, and the often-overlooked importance of controlling sodium and portion sizes. Additionally, we'll delve deeper into the powerful benefits of omega-3 fatty acids. Each section builds upon the last, helping you design an eating pattern that not only strengthens your heart but also enriches your emotional and mental well-being.

Harnessing the Power of Nutrient-Dense Foods

Why Nutrient Density Matters

Nutrient-dense foods are those that deliver **prominent levels of vitamins, minerals,** flavours, **and other beneficial compounds**, all while keeping calories, added sugars, and unhealthy fats relatively low. When your mainstay diet is built around these foods, you provide your heart with the essential building blocks it needs to perform optimally—every day, every hour, and every beat.

A heart-healthy diet does not have to mean bland. **Density** often comes hand in hand with vibrant colours, interesting textures, and delicious flavours. Think of the purple hue of blueberries, the bright orange of sweet potatoes, or the robust green of kale. These natural pigments not only make your plate visually appealing but also signify the presence of valuable antioxidants and phytochemicals that can protect the heart from damage.

The Antioxidant Advantage: Fruits and Vegetables

Fruits and vegetables rank among the most significant sources of antioxidants. These naturally occurring compounds neutralise harmful free radicals in your body, which can otherwise lead to oxidative stress – a critical factor in the development of cardiovascular disease.

- **Berries**: Blueberries, strawberries, raspberries, and blackberries are packed with vitamins, fibre, and antioxidants like anthocyanins, which may protect blood vessels.

- **Leafy Greens**: Spinach, kale, collard greens, and Swiss chard contain compounds such as lutein, folate, and magnesium—all essential for heart function and healthy blood pressure.

- **Tomatoes**: High in lycopene, tomatoes help maintain healthy cholesterol levels and may reduce the risk of stroke. Cooked tomatoes often provide more bioavailable lycopene than raw ones.

- **Cruciferous Vegetables**: Broccoli, cauliflower, and Brussels sprouts offer an array of nutrients while supporting detoxification processes in the body.

Incorporating fruits and vegetables into each meal can be as simple as adding spinach to your scrambled eggs, blending a cup of berries into your morning smoothie, or adding diced vegetables to your soups and stews. These small, consistent steps yield significant results over time, lowering inflammation and fortifying your cardiovascular system.

Whole Grains for Steady Energy and Cholesterol Control

Whole grains retain all parts of the grain kernel, including the bran, germ, and endosperm. This structure provides **fibre**, vitamins, and minerals that refined grains lack. Fibre plays a key role in lowering LDL (bad) cholesterol and improving HDL (good) cholesterol levels, reducing the burden on your heart.

Examples of whole grains include:

- **Oats**: A source of beta-glucan, soluble fibre that helps keep cholesterol in check.

- **Brown Rice**: Contains more fibre and nutrients than white rice, aiding in blood sugar regulation.

- **Quinoa**: A gluten-free option rich in protein, fibre, and minerals like magnesium and iron.

- **Barley**: High in soluble fibre, supports healthy cholesterol levels and digestion.

In addition to promoting heart health, whole grains offer steady, sustained energy by stabilising blood sugar. This is vital in preventing metabolic syndrome and type 2 diabetes, both of which increase cardiovascular risk. Replacing refined grains—like white bread or white pasta—with whole-grain equivalents can significantly reduce your chances of developing coronary artery disease.

Legumes: Versatile, Sustainable, and Heart-Healthy

Beans, lentils, and chickpeas belong to the legume family, offering a **low-fat, high-protein** alternative to meat. They are also loaded with fibre, vitamins, minerals, and antioxidants. Legumes help:

1. **Lower LDL Cholesterol**: Soluble fibre in beans binds to cholesterol in the digestive tract, ushering it out of the body.

2. **Regulate Blood Pressure**: Potassium and magnesium, prevalent in legumes, support normal blood pressure.

3. **Combat Inflammation**: Phytonutrients in legumes work to reduce systemic inflammation, a driving factor behind many heart conditions.

From lentil soups to bean-based stews, you can incorporate legumes in diverse, flavourful ways. Consider making a three-bean chilli or adding chickpeas to salads for a protein boost. For those who are environmentally conscious, legumes also have a lower carbon footprint compared to animal protein, thereby benefiting both your health and the planet.

Small Tweaks, Big Returns

These nutrient-dense foods fit seamlessly into most lifestyles. Simple swaps can include:

- Choosing **whole-grain** bread or pasta instead of refined versions.

- Snacking on **nuts and fruit** instead of chips or candy.

- Adding **extra vegetables** to casseroles, sandwiches and even sauces.

Each choice you make can bring you closer to a stronger, more resilient heart. The journey towards heart health often starts with these minor decisions – tiny steps that add up to lasting change.

Understanding Healthy Fats and Cholesterol

Decoding Dietary Fats

Not all fats have the same impact on your heart. Knowing the differences can help you consciously include heart-beneficial fats and limit detrimental ones.

1. **Saturated Fats**

   Primarily found in **animal products** (like red meat, butter, and cheese), as well as tropical oils (like coconut and palm oil), saturated fats can raise LDL cholesterol levels, increasing plaque buildup in arteries. While insignificant amounts can be part of a balanced diet, it is advisable to keep them in check, especially if you already have risk factors like high cholesterol, hypertension, or a family history of heart disease.

2. **Unsaturated Fats**

   These are considered **heart-friendly** because they help lower LDL while boosting HDL levels. Unsaturated fats come in 2 varieties: Both types have important roles in supporting healthy cholesterol levels and reducing inflammation. Swapping butter for olive oil, for instance, can help maintain a healthier lipid profile.

   - **Monounsaturated** (e.g., olive oil, avocados, certain nuts)

   - **Polyunsaturated** (e.g., sunflower oil, corn oil, fish)

3. **Trans Fats**

   Once widely used in processed foods and margarine for their extended shelf life, trans fats are the most harmful to heart health. They increase LDL and reduce HDL, significantly increasing the risk of coronary artery disease. Although regulatory measures have reduced trans fats in many countries, reading labels to avoid them remains crucial.

Why Triglycerides Matter

In addition to LDL and HDL cholesterol, triglycerides are another type of fat circulating in your bloodstream. When you consume **excess calories,** your body converts them into triglycerides and stores them in fat cells. High triglyceride levels can exacerbate your risk of heart disease and may signal issues such as:

- **Obesity**
- **Metabolic Syndrome**
- **Type 2 Diabetes**
- **Low Thyroid Function**

Lifestyle modifications – such as adopting a balanced diet, increasing physical activity, reducing alcohol intake, and maintaining a healthy weight – can help lower triglyceride levels and lighten the burden on your heart.

The Role of Cholesterol Transport: LDL vs. HDL

Cholesterol travels in the bloodstream via **lipoproteins**:

- **LDL (Low-Density Lipoprotein)**: Often called "bad" cholesterol, high LDL levels can lead to plaque formation in the arteries, impairing blood flow and increasing the risk of heart attacks and strokes.

- **HDL (High-Density Lipoprotein)**: Known as "good" cholesterol, it helps transport excess cholesterol back to the liver for recycling or excretion.

A balanced diet that prioritises **unsaturated fats**, along with regular exercise and stress management, can tip the balance towards higher HDL and lower LDL, providing significant cardiovascular protection.

Supercharging Your Diet with Healthy Fats

Seeds, nuts, and plant oils offer a rich spectrum of essential fatty acids, vitamins and minerals that help kerb inflammation. From chia seeds in your smoothie to pumpkin seeds sprinkled on salads, small additions can bring a wealth of benefits. Nut butters (like almond or peanut butter, provided they are minimally processed) can also be nutritious spreads or snack options.

When integrated sensibly, these healthy fats make meals more satisfying, reduce cravings for sugary snacks, and promote a stable energy supply—key for anyone juggling a busy schedule.

Incorporating Omega-3 Fatty Acids

Why Omega-3s Are Essential

Omega-3 fatty acids stand out for their extensive benefits. Because the human body **cannot** produce them, you must get them through your diet. The main types of omega-3s relevant to heart health include:

1. **EPA (Eicosapentaenoic Acid)**

2. **DHA (Docosahexaenoic Acid)**

3. **ALA (Alpha-Linolenic Acid)**

EPA and DHA, found primarily in **fatty fish**, are particularly effective at reducing triglyceride levels, maintaining normal blood pressure, and supporting the endothelium—the thin layer of cells that line your blood vessels. Meanwhile, ALA is found in **plant-based sources** like flaxseeds, walnuts, and chia seeds, though it must be converted into EPA and DHA in the body, a process that can be inefficient.

Omega-3 Benefits Beyond the Heart

In addition to lowering the risk of cardiovascular diseases, omega-3s:

- **Reduce Chronic Inflammation**: Inflammation contributes to numerous health problems, from joint pain to autoimmune conditions.

- **Improve Mental Health**: Studies suggest omega-3s can support cognitive function and alleviate symptoms of depression.

- **Strengthen Vision**: DHA is a structural component of the retina, and adequate intake may help maintain good eyesight.

Practical Ways to Boost Omega-3 Intake

- **Fatty Fish**: Salmon, mackerel, herring, and sardines are excellent sources. Aim for 2 servings (around 3.5 ounces each) per week.

- **Plant-Based Options**: For vegetarians or vegans, include flaxseeds, chia seeds, hemp seeds, and walnuts regularly. Consider speaking with a healthcare provider about algae-based DHA supplements if needed.

- **Recipe Ideas:**
    - ☐ Top salads or oatmeal with ground flaxseeds or chia seeds.
    - ☐ Use chopped walnuts for a crunchy texture on roasted vegetables.
    - ☐ Replace red meat with salmon fillets at least a couple of times a week.

Supplements: A Cautious Approach

For some individuals—especially those with high triglycerides or specific heart conditions—**omega-3 supplements** (like fish oil capsules) may provide additional benefits. However, it is essential to consult a healthcare professional before starting any supplement. Certain formulations may interact with medications or be contraindicated for certain conditions. Personalised guidance will help you find the correct dosage, if necessary, and manage any risks.

Reducing Sodium: A Vital Step for Heart Health

The Sodium-Blood Pressure Connection

Excess sodium can be a silent saboteur of heart health. Consuming more sodium than your body needs contribute to **high blood pressure** (hypertension), a leading risk factor for heart disease and stroke. Blood pressure rises because too much sodium disrupts the kidney's ability to remove water, increasing fluid in the bloodstream and forcing the heart to work harder.

The recommended daily sodium intake for most adults is **2,300 mg or less**, but many people regularly exceed this, often without realising it. Processed foods—like deli meats, frozen meals, canned soups, and fast-food—are typically loaded with sodium to enhance flavour and extend shelf life.

Strategies for Managing Sodium Intake

- **Cook at Home**: Preparing fresh meals allows you to control ingredients. Season foods with herbs, spices, lemon juice, or vinegar to add flavour without extra salt.

- **Label Literacy**: Always check nutrition labels for sodium content. Terms like "low-sodium," "no salt added," and "reduced sodium" can guide healthier choices. Compare brands to find the option with the least sodium.

- **Mindful Dining Out**: Request less salt when ordering restaurant meals. Many chefs can accommodate this. Opt for sauces and dressings on the side so you can manage how much you use.

- **Rinse Canned Foods**: Rinsing canned beans or vegetables can significantly reduce their sodium content, making them a more heart-friendly option.

Even small, consistent reductions in sodium can **noticeably lower blood pressure**. Over time, your taste buds adjust, and you may even start to find processed, salty foods overwhelming.

Overcoming Barriers to Sodium Reduction

Social gatherings, holiday feasts, and busy work schedules can make low-sodium eating feel challenging. However, with **planning and adaptation**, it is feasible—and rewarding. For instance:

- **Batch Cooking**: Prepare low-sodium meals in large batches during the weekend. Freeze them in individual portions for quick meals throughout the week.

- **Spice Blends**: Experiment with cultural spice mixes (e.g., Indian, Mediterranean, or Cajun) that can bring out new dimensions of flavour without relying heavily on salt.

- **At Work**: Keep healthy, low-sodium snacks (like unsalted nuts, fresh fruits, or low-sodium crackers) at your desk. This practice can prevent vending machine or fast-food temptations during busy days.

Reducing sodium not only protects your heart but also often leads to greater overall health, **including more stable energy levels, a better mood, and improved kidney function.** For families, a collective commitment to reducing sodium can reinforce healthy habits for children from an early age, establishing a pattern they can carry into adulthood.

Mastering Portion Control

Why Portion Sizes Matter

Even the healthiest foods, when eaten in excess, can contribute to weight gain and metabolic stress. Modern food environments—like oversized restaurant portions and "value meals"—have normalised larger servings. Over time, our perception of what constitutes a **normal portion** has become distorted.

Weight gain, in turn, can lead to **high blood pressure**, elevated cholesterol, and a higher risk of type 2 diabetes. Each of these factors can strain the heart. Mastering portion control does not mean deprivation; it is about aligning with your body's genuine nutritional needs.

Practical Tips for Perfect Portion Sizes

1. **Use Smaller Plates and Bowls**

   A visually full small plate is more satisfying than a half-empty large plate, thanks to psychological cues that influence satiety.

2. **Measure It Out**

   Kitchen tools like measuring cups, spoons, and food scales help you understand actual serving sizes. This step is particularly helpful during the initial stages of adopting healthier habits.

3. **Portion Control Plates**

   Many companies produce plates divided into sections for **vegetables, proteins, and starches.** These tools offer simple, visual guideline, especially useful for families teaching children about balanced meals.

4. **Mindful Eating**

Focus on each flavour and texture. Put down your fork between bites and listen to your body's hunger and fullness signals. This mindful approach helps prevent overeating and fosters a healthier relationship with food.

Overcoming Challenges to Portion Control

- **Social Settings**: In some cultures, or family traditions, substantial portions are synonymous with generosity and hospitality. You can politely decline seconds or ask for a smaller serving initially, explaining that you want to ensure you do not waste food or overeat.

- **Emotional Eating**: Stress, boredom, and sadness can trigger mindless snacking. Recognise these triggers and find alternative coping strategies, such as going for a walk, meditating, or listening to music.

- **Restaurant Meals**: Restaurants often serve more than one portion's worth of food on a single plate. Consider sharing an entrée or boxing up half of your meal before you start eating.

Over time, these strategies recalibrate your concept of a **reasonable serving size**, supporting better weight management and heart health. For families, working together to standardise portion sizes at mealtimes can create consistency, reduce tension around food choices, and foster an environment where everyone learns to appreciate quality over quantity.

Emotional and Social Aspects of Heart-Healthy Eating

The Joy of Cooking and Sharing Meals

One of the most overlooked elements of heart-healthy eating is the **emotional satisfaction** it can bring. Cooking is not just about following recipes – it can be an act of love, creativity, and self-care. Exploring new spices, ingredients, and techniques can spark excitement and help you view food preparation as a positive, life-affirming activity.

Family meals can have profound emotional benefits. Studies indicate that **eating together** fosters better communication, stronger family bonds, and healthier eating patterns in children. Sitting down as a family or with friends, free from electronic devices, allows for deeper connections and mindful eating. This is especially important given the stress and isolation that many people face in modern life.

Involving Children in Healthy Choices

For those with children, it is crucial to **model behaviours** early. Kids who learn about nutrient-dense foods and portion sizes at an early age often continue those habits later in life. Simple ways to involve them include:

- Letting them help with **meal prep**, such as washing vegetables or mixing ingredients.

- Teaching them to **read food labels**, emphasising the importance of checking for sodium, added sugars, and trans fats.

- Encouraging them to **taste test new foods**, turning healthy eating into a fun adventure.

By involving children in decision-making, you empower them to take ownership of their food choices, which can set them up for a lifetime of nutritional awareness and heart-conscious living.

Cultural and Social Celebrations

From holiday feasts to community potlucks, food plays a significant role in cultural and social gatherings. Adopting heart-healthy practices does not mean you must abstain from celebrations or drastically alter traditional dishes. Instead, you can:

- **Adjust Recipes**: Use healthier cooking methods (baking, steaming, grilling) rather than frying. Reduce salt and sugar incrementally, substituting herbs, spices, citrus, or vinegar for flavour.

- **Balanced Serving**: Enjoy your favourite indulgent dishes in moderation while filling most of your plate with nutrient-dense salads, vegetables, or fruits.

- **Encourage Healthy Potluck Contributions**: Offer to bring a heart-friendly dish to share, such as a vegetable-based casserole or a fruit salad. This ensures there's a nutritious option at the table for everyone.

These strategies help ensure that your social life remains rich and enjoyable while you continue to prioritise cardiovascular well-being.

Overcoming Obstacles and Maintaining Momentum

Common Pitfalls

1. **All-or-Nothing Thinking** All-or-nothing thinking

2. **Relying on Quick Fixes**: Trendy diets or detoxes might promise dramatic results, but they often neglect the complexity of true heart health. Sustainable lifestyle changes trump extreme dietary approaches.

3. **Underestimating Hidden Ingredients**: Assorted condiments, sauces, and dressings can add hidden sodium, sugar, and unhealthy fats. Be mindful of nutritional labels, even for items that seem benign.

Staying Motivated Over the Long Haul

- **Set Realistic Goals**: Aim for small, attainable milestones, such as eating fruit or vegetable with every meal or cooking one new healthy recipe per week.

- **Track Your Progress**: Use a food journal, mobile app, or wearable device to track your dietary habits, water intake, and physical activity. Tracking can highlight areas for improvement and reinforce positive changes.

- **Celebrate Wins**: Whether it is lower blood pressure, weight loss, or simply feeling more energetic, acknowledge and celebrate your progress. Rewards can be non-food items—like a new workout outfit or a relaxing massage.

- **Find Support**: Work with a dietitian, join a heart health support group, or pair up with a friend or family member who shares your goals. Mutual accountability can make all the difference.

Final Thoughts

Understanding how nutrition shapes heart health is a cornerstone of **lifelong well-being**. Each chapter in this journey underscores that the power to protect and nurture your heart lies in your hands—and on your plate. By choosing **antioxidant-rich fruits and vegetables, whole grains**, and **legumes**, you supply your cardiovascular system with the nutrients it needs to function optimally. Recognising the differences among saturated, unsaturated, and trans fats allows you to make informed choices that favour healthy cholesterol levels. Embracing the benefits of **omega-3 fatty acids** further boosts inflammation reduction and overall vitality.

Stepping back from high-sodium foods can guard against hypertension, a silent but formidable threat to heart health. Meanwhile, mastering **portion control** ensures that you avoid the hidden pitfalls of excess calories, even if those calories come from healthier sources. Along the way, it is equally important to acknowledge the emotional and cultural dimensions of eating, which can either nurture or undermine your progress. Cooking and sharing meals with loved ones can become a source of joy, bonding, and collective commitment.

A heart-healthy lifestyle does not demand perfection. It asks for **awareness, consistency, and resilience** in the face of temptations and obstacles. When you slip—and everyone does—kindness towards yourself is key. Each meal offers a new opportunity to course-correct and recommit. As you adopt these dietary strategies and integrate them into your daily routine, you will notice benefits that reach well beyond your heart. Better sleep, improved mood, heightened energy levels, and a more robust immune system often follow a healthy eating pattern.

Your Call to Action

- **Reflect**: Take a moment to consider the areas of your diet that may need attention. What does your current plate look like, and where can you add more fibre, antioxidants, and healthy fats?

- **Act**: Identify one or 2 specific changes you can make this week—such as replacing a refined grain with a whole-grain, committing to 2 servings of fish, or cutting back on salty processed snacks.

- **Assess**: Over the next month, note how these changes affect your energy levels, waistline, mood, and any relevant health markers like blood pressure or cholesterol. Share your successes and challenges with a supportive friend or family member.

- **Iterate**: Heart health is a lifelong journey, and your dietary habits will evolve. Remain open to experimenting with new foods, recipes, and cooking methods that keep your meals both nutritious and exciting.

By weaving these habits into your everyday life, you gift yourself—and those around you—**the promise of a healthier tomorrow**. Good nutrition is an investment in your future, a testament to the value you place on living fully and well. As you continue reading this book and applying its principles, remember that the power of change lies within you. Each meal is a chance to fortify your heart, energise your body, and embrace a richer, more vibrant life.

Push Your Pulse:
How Staying Active Fuels a Healthier Heart

Physical Activity: The Heart's Most Loyal Ally

The human heart is nothing short of a miracle - an enduring engine that pumps blood every second of every day to sustain life. Yet, in the hustle and bustle of modern existence, we often overlook the significance of caring for this vital organ. We rely on it to keep beating faithfully, but do we offer anything in return?

One of the most direct, impactful ways to nurture your heart is through **physical activity**. Regular exercise is about more than sculpting a fit physique or shedding extra pounds. It is an investment in your heart's strength, your body's resilience, and your mental well-being. By embracing an active lifestyle, you can reduce the risk of cardiovascular diseases, invigorate your daily energy levels, and experience the emotional rewards that come from caring for your body.

This journey is not just for solo adventurers. Families can transform exercise into a bonding activity, creating cherished memories and lifelong habits. Young adults stepping into newfound independence can make active living a cornerstone of their self-care routine. Regardless of age or fitness level, physical activity can become the foundation for a life lived with greater vigour, mental clarity, and, of course, heart health.

In this chapter, we'll explore the essential role of exercise in promoting cardiovascular wellness. From building a personalised routine to overcoming common barriers, you will find practical steps to ensure that your pursuit of fitness becomes both sustainable and deeply rewarding.

The Foundation of Fitness: Designing a Personalised Plan

1. Assess Your Starting Point

Every successful journey begins with understanding where you stand. Before delving into workouts and schedules, it is wise to evaluate your current fitness level. Doing so prevents overexertion, reduces the risk of injury, and allows you to set realistic expectations.

- **Aerobic Capacity:** Take note of how long or how far you can walk, jog, or cycle without feeling overly fatigued. This will be your baseline for cardiovascular endurance.

- **Muscle Strength:** Simple bodyweight exercises like push-ups, squats, or sit-ups provide insight into your overall strength. Count how many repetitions you can manage while maintaining proper form.

- **Flexibility:** Touching your toes or performing basic stretches can reveal areas of tightness. Improving flexibility makes all types of exercise more accessible and comfortable.

- **Balance:** Standing on one foot or doing a heel-to-toe walk can show whether your sense of balance and core strength needs work.

Some people opt for professional assessments—like VO_2 max tests, body composition scans, or supervised exercise stress tests—to get detailed metrics. While these can be helpful, they are not always necessary. Even a self-guided evaluation can be enough to set you on the right path.

2. Recognise Personal Boundaries

It is important to remember that no 2 bodies are exactly alike. Past injuries, chronic health conditions, and genetic factors all influence what types of exercise are best for you. If you have had knee surgery, for example, you might benefit from water aerobics or stationary biking instead of high-impact running. Those living with arthritis may find yoga or gentle Pilates more comfortable and beneficial.

For individuals with existing cardiovascular risks—like high blood pressure, high cholesterol, or a history of heart disease—consultation with a healthcare provider is crucial. A doctor or certified trainer can help you devise a routine that challenges you safely. Exercising wisely means balancing ambition with respect for your body's limits, ensuring that each movement is both beneficial and secure.

3. Find Activities That Spark Joy

Consistency is the secret ingredient to long-term fitness, and the best way to stay consistent is to truly enjoy what you are doing. Think back to hobbies that brought you joy—it was dancing, hiking, riding a bike, or even roller-skating. Integrating these activities into your weekly routine transforms "working out" into an eagerly anticipated pastime.

Many find that group classes, such as Zumba or spin sessions, offer a supportive environment brimming with motivation. Others may prefer a quiet nature trail for jogging or walking, where they can reflect and relieve stress. The key is to experiment and discover an exercise style that resonates. When workouts are pleasurable, you will be far less likely to skip them, leading to sustainable progress over time.

4. Create a Balanced Routine

A comprehensive fitness plan typically includes 3 core components:

1. **Cardiovascular Exercise:** Activities that elevate your heart rate and challenge your endurance—like brisk walking, swimming, dancing, or jogging.

2. **Strength Training:** Exercises that build muscle mass and bone density, such as weightlifting, bodyweight workouts, or resistance band movements.

3. **Flexibility and Balance Training:** Stretches, yoga poses, or balance drills that foster mobility, reduce injury risks, and support functional movement.

Your schedule should weave these elements together in a way that suits your lifestyle. Here is a sample structure to consider:

- **Monday & Thursday:** Cardiovascular exercises (e.g., brisk walking, cycling, or dance workouts).

- **Tuesday & Friday:** Strength training (e.g., weightlifting, resistance bands, or bodyweight exercises).

- **Wednesday & Saturday:** Flexibility and balance (e.g., yoga, Pilates, or dedicated stretching sessions).

- **Sunday:** Rest or light activity (e.g., leisurely strolls, gentle swimming, or family sports day).

The American Heart Association recommends at least **150 minutes of moderate aerobic exercise** or **75 minutes of vigorous aerobic exercise** per week. This can be broken into small increments—like 3 10-minute walks a day—to accommodate busy schedules. Adding at least **2 strength training sessions** per week targets major muscle groups and amplifies cardiovascular benefits. Lastly, consider dedicating even a brief period each day to stretching or balancing drills, ensuring a well-rounded approach.

The Cardiovascular Cornerstone

1. What Are Cardiovascular Exercises?

Cardiovascular (or aerobic) exercises are workouts that ramp up your heart rate and breathing, prompting your heart and lungs to work more strenuously. By increasing oxygen demand, your body adapts over time, making you more capable of everyday tasks and less prone to fatigue.

Examples of Cardiovascular Exercises:

- **Walking or Jogging:** A simple, low-cost option suitable for beginners.

- **Swimming:** The water's buoyancy reduces impact on joints, making it excellent for people with arthritis or joint pain.

- **Cycling:** Stationary bikes or outdoor rides help build endurance.

- **Dancing:** Whether it is salsa, line dancing, or a Zumba class, dancing mixes fun, social interaction, and cardio all in one.

- **HIIT (High-Intensity Interval Training):** Short bursts of intense activity followed by rest intervals; highly effective for boosting cardiovascular fitness in a limited time.

2. Heart Health and Beyond

While cardiovascular exercise undeniably strengthens your heart, its benefits spill into multiple facets of life:

- **Improved Circulation:** A robust heart pumps blood more effectively, ensuring that organs and muscles receive adequate oxygen and nutrients.

- **Blood Pressure and Cholesterol Management:** Regular cardio is associated with lower blood pressure, reduced LDL (bad) cholesterol, and elevated HDL (good) cholesterol levels.

- **Weight Control:** Aerobic activities burn calories, aiding in weight management. This relieves extra strain on the heart and helps prevent obesity-related conditions.

- **Mood Boost and Mental Clarity:** Exercise triggers the release of endorphins—often called "feel-good" hormones—that can alleviate stress, reduce anxiety, and improve mental focus.

From staving off chronic diseases to enhancing your day-to-day vitality, consistent cardiovascular exercise is a linchpin in a healthy lifestyle.

3. Making Cardio a Daily Habit

Turning cardiovascular activity into a non-negotiable part of your routine does not have to be daunting:

- **Start Small:** If you are new to exercise, aim for short, 10- to 15-minute sessions and gradually increase duration and intensity.

- **Combine Tasks:** Walk or cycle to work or squeeze in a few brisk laps around the car park during lunch breaks.

- **Social Approach:** Join a local running club, participate in charity walks, or invite friends for weekend hikes—shared goals heighten accountability.

- **Stay Flexible:** Life is full of surprises. If you miss a morning jog, try a 20-minute walk after dinner or dance along to a home workout video.

As you rack up small victories, your stamina and confidence will grow, fuelling a positive cycle that keeps you engaged and excited about continued improvement.

Building Strength for a Healthy Heart

1. Why Strength Training Matters

When people think of heart health, they often gravitate towards images of treadmills and jogging shoes. Yet, **strength training** is equally vital for a balanced regimen. Adding muscle mass not only shapes a more toned physique but also alleviates cardiovascular strain. Greater muscle mass translates into a higher basal metabolic rate, meaning you burn more calories—even when at rest.

Additionally, stronger muscles support better posture, improve joint stability, and make other exercises more effective. Over time, enhancing muscular strength also bolsters endurance. If you can lift heavier objects or sustain a plank for longer, you will discover that tasks like climbing stairs, gardening, or playing with your kids become less taxing on your body and your heart.

2. The Benefits of Strength Training

- **Cardiovascular Support:** Muscle development and aerobic performance go hand in hand, enabling your heart to handle incremental increases in activity.

- **Bone Health:** Resistance exercises, including bodyweight workouts and free weights, stimulate bone growth and density, significantly lowering the risk of fractures and osteoporosis.

- **Functional Fitness:** Everyday tasks—such as carrying groceries, picking up children, or engaging in recreational sports—become more manageable when your muscles are robust, and your core is stable.

3. Getting Started with Strength Training

If you are unaccustomed to lifting weights, gradual progression is key to avoiding injuries and burnout.

- **Bodyweight Basics:** Begin with push-ups, squats, lunges, and planks—these exercises require no equipment and can be adapted to various fitness levels.

- **Resistance Bands or Machines:** For those seeking more variety, try incorporating resistance bands or weight machines at a gym. Both provide support and help you isolate different muscle groups.

- **Free Weights:** Dumbbells and kettlebells offer versatile options as you gain confidence. Start with lighter weights and focus on form, eventually increasing the load or volume when it feels too easy.

- **Frequency and Progression:** Aim for 2 strength training sessions per week, targeting all major muscle groups (legs, back, core, arms, chest, and shoulders). As you become more proficient, increase the intensity—adding extra sets, heavier weights, or more challenging variations.

A qualified personal trainer can be a game-changer when it comes to designing a programme tailored to your goals. They can demonstrate proper techniques, suggest appropriate progressions, and ensure you are consistently working within safe boundaries.

Flexibility and Balance: The Unsung Heroes

1. The Role of Flexibility

Flexibility is a sometimes-overlooked component of fitness, yet it plays a critical role in injury prevention and functional movement. When your muscles and connective tissues can stretch adequately, your body can move more gracefully, and you reduce unnecessary strain on your joints.

Regular stretching sessions, be they dynamic (gentle movement-based stretches) or static (holding a position for a set period), can improve posture and range of motion. Over time, this contributes to better workouts in other fitness domains—cardio and strength training both become more fluid and safer when you are not hindered by tightness.

2. Benefits of Balance

Balance is another cornerstone of physical well-being, though it is often taken for granted until issues arise. For older adults, a strong balance can help prevent falls and potentially life-altering injuries. Younger and middle-aged individuals benefit too—enhanced balance translating smoother athletic performance in sports and daily tasks alike.

Core-focused exercises, such as planks, Pilates routines, and single-leg movements, train the body to stabilise itself effectively. Even brief sessions can yield significant improvements, such as feeling more secure when navigating uneven terrain or carrying heavy objects.

3. How to Incorporate Flexibility and Balance

- **Yoga and Pilates:** These practice styles merge stretching, balance, and mindfulness. Yoga postures (asanas) gently open tight areas, while Pilates emphasises core strength and controlled movements.

- **Post-Workout Stretches:** Finish each exercise session with a dedicated stretch routine targeting key muscle groups such as calves, hamstrings, quads, and shoulders.

- **Simple Balance Drills:** Standing on one foot, walking in a straight-line heel-to-toe, or using a wobble board are effortless ways to hone stability.

- **Consistency Over Perfection:** A few minutes of stretching and balancing each day can add up to powerful, long-lasting benefits, so do not underestimate short but focused sessions.

Overcoming Barriers to Staying Active

Even the most well-intentioned plans can be disrupted by life's various roadblocks. Time limitations, waning motivation, and juggling family schedules are just a few familiar challenges. Recognising these hurdles—and preparing strategies to tackle them—can keep you from derailing your newfound commitment to fitness.

1. Time Constraints

Our modern world often operates at breakneck speed, leaving little time for leisurely pursuits. However, if something is important enough, we find ways to prioritise it. Here are a few strategies to weave exercise into a busy life:

- **Micro-Workouts:** Opt for short bursts of activity—such as 10-minute walks or 5-minute strength circuits—spread throughout the day. Over time, these mini-sessions add up.

- **Active Commutes:** If feasible, walk or cycle to work, run errands on foot, or park farther away when driving.

- **Efficient Routines:** High-intensity interval training (HIIT) provides an effective workout in a compressed timeframe. Combine strength and cardio in a circuit to maximise results.

2. Lack of Motivation

Motivation can ebb and flow. The initial excitement of starting a new programme might wane as weeks pass, and progress sometimes seems slow. To counteract this:

- **Set Clear, Incremental Goals:** Instead of vague targets like "get fit," aim for objectives such as "run for 10 minutes without stopping" or "increase squat reps from 10 to 20 over a month." Concrete goals maintain momentum.

- **Track Achievements:** Journals, apps, or wearable devices can document gains in distance, strength, or consistency, offering tangible proof of success.

- **Join a Community:** Consider local sports leagues, gym classes, or online forums where members share triumphs and offer support. Friendships built around shared fitness goals can be a powerful motivator.

3. Family Involvement

For many, balancing the demands of parenthood or caring for relatives leaves little room for personal workouts. Yet, turning fitness into a **family affair** can solve multiple issues at once:

- **Weekend Adventures:** Organise hikes, bike rides, or backyard soccer matches that blend fun and exercise for all ages.

- **Household Routines:** Encourage everyone to join a daily post-dinner walk or an early morning stretching session. This fosters unity and makes being an active part of family culture.

- **Child Participation:** Let kids mimic simple exercises or set up obstacle courses. They will burn energy, and you will sneak in a workout—win-win.

Tracking Progress and Sustaining Success

Success in fitness—especially for heart health—relies on consistency and a willingness to adapt. Monitoring your journey helps you notice improvements you might otherwise overlook and provides a roadmap for future goals.

1. The Power of Progress Tracking

Whether you opt for smartphone apps, paper journals, or wearable fitness trackers, logging your workouts can reveal patterns and improvements. You might notice that your jogging pace quickens or that you feel stronger doing push-ups. These insights validate your efforts and can reignite your drive when motivation dips.

2. Celebrating Milestones

Every victory, no matter how seemingly small, merits celebration. Did you walk for 30 consecutive minutes for the first time? Did you achieve a new personal best in squats? Recognising achievements can take many forms:

- **Rewards:** Treat yourself to new workout gear, a relaxing massage, or a healthy cookbook.

- **Sharing with Others:** Post your progress on social media or update friends and family. A sense of communal pride in your efforts can be a potent incentive.

- **Personal Reflection:** Maintain a journal where you jot down how each success makes you feel. Over time, you will build a record of positive transformations—physically, mentally, and emotionally.

3. Staying Adaptable

Routines that remain static are more prone to becoming stale. Once your body adapts, you may hit a plateau where progress stalls. If this happens, mix things up:

- **Vary Intensity:** Increase weights, speed up your running pace, or add short sprints to your usual cycling route.

- **Explore New Activities:** If you have been jogging outdoors, try a dance class or yoga workshop. Alternate strength training days with different techniques, such as kettlebell circuits or TRX suspension exercises.

- **Set Fresh Goals:** If your original milestone was to walk 10,000 steps daily, push it to 12,000 or incorporate a weekly 5K run. By continually challenging yourself, you keep your workouts mentally engaging and physically effective.

4. Embracing Periodisation

Serious athletes swear by a concept called "periodisation," which involves dividing training into cycles—each focusing on different goals, intensities, or styles of exercise. While you might not be an Olympic contender, borrowing this principle can help avoid overtraining and support systematic growth. For instance, you might spend 4–6 weeks emphasising endurance, followed by a phase concentrating on strength, then transition to agility and core stabilisation. These structured changes prevent monotony and injuries while allowing your body to adapt in new ways.

The Emotional and Social Dimensions of Exercise

A comprehensive view of fitness goes beyond physical. Exercise also acts as a bridge to emotional well-being and social connections. By acknowledging these intangible aspects, you can anchor your fitness journey in a sense of meaning and belonging.

1. Mental Health Benefits

Numerous studies link regular physical activity to mental health benefits:

- **Stress Relief:** Exercise helps lower levels of cortisol, a hormone linked to stress and anxiety.

- **Enhanced Mood:** A rush of endorphins during workouts can combat mild depression and elevate your overall sense of contentment.

- **Better Sleep:** Engaging in moderate activity can regulate sleep cycles, helping you fall asleep faster and enjoy deeper rest.

2. Social Connections

Fitness does not have to be a solitary pursuit. Joining a local running club, gym class, or sports team introduces you to people with shared interests. Whether it is a group of hikers exploring local trails each weekend or an after-work basketball league, these communal experiences can enrich your social life and provide another layer of accountability.

3. Family Bonds

Exercising as a family encourages teamwork and communication. Children exposed to healthy role models at home are more likely to adopt and retain active habits into adulthood. Plus, the memories formed while conquering a hiking trail together or practising yoga in the living room can become cherished family stories, reinforcing bonds through shared accomplishment.

Addressing Special Populations and Life Stages

Every stage of life presents unique challenges and opportunities for physical activity. By tailoring approaches for different ages and circumstances, you can ensure that everyone's journey remains safe, relevant, and engaging.

1. Children and Adolescents

For kids, movement is often a by-product of play. Encouraging them to participate in sports, dance, or just active games is crucial for their overall development. Physical activity supports healthy growth of bones and muscles, improves coordination, and sets the stage for a lifelong positive relationship with exercise. However, avoid imposing rigorous training regimens. Instead, emphasise **fun** and exploration, allowing them to discover athletic passions naturally.

2. Young Adults

Stepping into independence, be it college, a career, or living on your own—offers a prime window to establish lifelong habits. If you can weave regular workouts into your routine during these formative years, you will be more likely to keep them up amid future life changes. Additionally, initiative-taking cardiovascular fitness in your 20s and 30s can significantly reduce the risk of heart disease later.

3. Middle-Aged Adults

Balancing demanding jobs, family responsibilities, and community obligations can leave this group strapped for time. Short, high-intensity workouts or flexible home-based routines may be ideal solutions. Staying active helps manage weight gain often experienced in middle age and combats rising health risks such as hypertension, elevated cholesterol, and type 2 diabetes.

4. Older Adults

The golden years bring specific considerations, such as reduced bone density, potential joint issues, and a slower recovery rate. However, consistent physical activity remains vital. Lower-impact exercises like swimming, light resistance training, and gentle yoga can maintain joint mobility, preserve muscle mass, and improve balance—key factors in preventing falls. Always consult healthcare providers for personalised guidance and to adapt routines, as necessary.

5. Individuals with Chronic Conditions

For those managing conditions like diabetes, obesity, or heart disease, exercise can be an integral part of treatment. Under medical guidance, moderate activities (e.g., brisk walking, chair exercises) can help control blood sugar, reduce inflammation, and improve cardiovascular markers. Collaboration with doctors or physical therapists ensures you select exercises that are safe yet effective, enabling steady progress without risking complications.

Final Thoughts: Embrace an Active Lifestyle

Physical activity is one of the most profound gifts you can offer your heart and entire body. It is an ongoing conversation between your mind, muscles, and cardiovascular system—a dynamic interplay that evolves as you gain strength and resilience. Through consistent movement, you can prevent or mitigate chronic health issues, maintain emotional balance, and discover the joys of pushing your boundaries.

As you navigate the twists and turns of life, remember:

1. **Start Where You Are**: There's no requirement to be an athlete. Simply commit to consistent small steps, whether walking around the block, dancing in your living room, or trying a new gym class.

2. **Respect Your Body**: Listen to cues like pain or excessive fatigue. Progress should be gradual, building upon your existing capabilities without overwhelming them.

3. **Seek Joy**: When exercise is fun, it becomes a cherished part of your day. Explore a variety of activities to find what resonates most deeply.

4. **Adapt and Grow**: Your fitness needs will shift over time. Stay flexible—literally and figuratively—and remain open to changing your routine as your lifestyle evolves.

5. **Celebrate Milestones**: From small victories like mastering a new yoga pose to major achievements like completing a 5K, every success is a testament to your perseverance.

By weaving movement into the fabric of your day—step by step, choice by choice—you create a life that celebrates vitality, connection, and well-being. Each brisk walk you take, each minute spent strengthening muscles, and each yoga pose you hold sends a signal to your heart: *I appreciate you.* Indeed, your heart is your most loyal ally, and physical activity is among the simplest yet most powerful ways to repay its unwavering devotion.

No matter where you stand right now—whether in youth or advanced age, as a busy parent or a single adult—the decision to prioritise physical activity can reshape your health trajectory. Welcome it as a companion for the journey, a source of empowerment that transforms your heart's performance, your sense of self, and your outlook on life.

You have the tools; this chapter lays out the map. The next move is yours to make. Embrace an active lifestyle and give your heart the gratitude it deserves—one step, one rep, one breath at a time.

Rest and Recharge:
Stress Relief for a Healthy Heart

Mastering Stress Management for Heart Health

Stress can be an insidious part of modern life, creeping into your thoughts, routines, and relationships without warning. It might begin as a mere annoyance—like rushing to meet a deadline or dealing with a family disagreement—but it can escalate into chronic tension that undermines physical and mental well-being. Regarding heart health, stress is pivotal in influencing blood pressure, heart rate, and overall cardiovascular function. Yet, while the connection between stress and heart health can be significant, it does not have to be a life sentence.

This chapter explores how effectively managing stress protects the heart from undue strain and enriches your daily life. You will learn to identify the subtle and overt stress triggers, adopt mindfulness and relaxation strategies, curate a home environment that promotes serenity, and develop healthy coping mechanisms that foster resilience. Families, young adults, and anyone else aiming to safeguard their heart health will discover valuable insights on weaving stress management seamlessly into everyday routines.

Identifying Sources of Stress

Understanding the Hidden Undercurrent of Stress

Stress often functions like an undercurrent—unnoticed at first, only intensifying until it disrupts emotional and physical stability. Whether it is a buildup of minor daily irritations or a singular overwhelming event, unmanaged stress can drive your body into a state of heightened alert, known as the fight-or-flight response. Over time, chronic stress may elevate your risk of hypertension, heart disease, and other health complications.

Identifying what triggers this harmful cycle is the first step in dismantling it. Pinpointing your stressors involves keen self-awareness and a commitment to self-examination, akin to becoming a detective of your own life. By uncovering the root causes—work demands, family conflict, financial worries, or health concerns, you move towards designing effective strategies to cope with them.

Journaling: A Window into Daily Struggles

Journaling is a simple yet powerful way to spot stress patterns. Writing down your thoughts, feelings, and experiences at the end of each day helps you reflect on events that might otherwise blur together. You consistently note irritations during your morning commute or anxiety spikes whenever you have a work meeting. Over time, a journal reveals recurring triggers and highlights the cumulative effect of small stressors.

Research by Falon et al. (2022) indicates that people often overlook how minor pressures accrue over time. You may not recall any standout stressors when asked how your week went, yet journaling can reveal a hidden buildup of tension—like a slow drip adding up in a bucket until it overflows.

Practical Tip: Dedicate 5–10 minutes each evening to write down the day's notable events, emotions, and physical symptoms. Pay particular attention to patterns of frustration, anxiety, or fatigue. Identifying these patterns creates a roadmap for addressing or eliminating them.

Self-Assessment Tools and Conversations

In addition to journaling, various **self-assessment tools**—such as smartphone apps, mood trackers, or online questionnaires—can help you better understand your emotional responses. These tools systematically collect data on your mood shifts, highlighting correlations between specific circumstances and emotional highs or lows.

Another often overlooked method is talking with trusted friends or family. Loved ones may see signs of stress you are too close to recognise. A candid conversation invites an external perspective, which can help you spot triggers or confirm suspicions about certain stressors. This open dialogue nurtures strong social bonds, creating a sense of shared understanding and support.

When to Seek Professional Guidance

Chronic stress can be especially damaging, masking itself as a "normal" routine yet steadily taxing your emotional and physical resources. If you suspect that long-term stress has become ingrained—manifesting through insomnia, recurring anxiety, irritability, or physical ailments—it may be time to consult a mental health professional. Therapists, counsellors, or healthcare providers possess the expertise to uncover hidden triggers, suggest coping strategies, and guide you towards healthier thought patterns.

Key Takeaway: Identifying sources of stress is more than an intellectual exercise; it is a foundational skill for overall well-being. Individuals and families can expose the hidden triggers that erode heart health by systematically tracking emotional responses via journaling, self-assessment tools, or discussions. Gaining this awareness is the first step in forming meaningful and lasting stress management techniques.

Practising Mindfulness and Meditation

Why Mindfulness Matters for Heart Health

Mindfulness is the practice of remaining fully present in the moment, a gentle discipline of observing thoughts, emotions, and bodily sensations without judgement. In our fast-paced world—marked by perpetual to do lists and digital distractions—this ancient concept has emerged scientifically for modern stress. Chronic stress stimulates the release of cortisol, a hormone that can increase heart rate, blood pressure, and inflammation when elevated for extended periods.

Adopting mindfulness is not about disconnecting from reality or ignoring responsibilities. Rather, it is about **shifting how you respond** to life's pressures. By cultivating presence, you break the cycle of dwelling on past regrets or fretting about future uncertainties—both of which can perpetuate stress.

Breath Awareness

A foundational mindfulness exercise is **breath awareness**, a technique that harnesses the natural rhythm of breathing to anchor the mind. Here is how it works:

1. **Find a Quiet Space**: Sit comfortably, close your eyes, and allow the tension in your shoulders and jaw to dissolve.

2. **Observe Your Breath**: Notice each inhale and exhale, feeling the cool air entering your nostrils and the warm air exiting.

3. **Refocus When Drifting**: Inevitably, thoughts will pop up. Rather than wrestling with them, gently return your focus to your breath each time you notice your mind has wandered.

This simple practice, even for just a few minutes daily, can recalibrate an overactive response to stress. Over time, breath awareness can lower resting heart rates, stabilise blood pressure, and promote a calm mental state.

Guided Meditations and Body Scans

Guided meditations provide structured support, especially for beginners unsure how to quiet the mental chatter. Through audio or video, an instructor leads you through visualisation and breathing exercises step by step. Examples include imagery of a peaceful lakeside or a forest walk, helping you gradually release pent-up anxiety.

Meanwhile, the **body scan technique** systematically directs attention through various parts of your body. Begin at your toes and progress upward, noticing any tension or discomfort. This process not only alleviates physical stress but also sharpens self-awareness. Acknowledging where stress manifests in your body empowers you to release it consciously.

Mindful Movements: Yoga and More

For those craving a physical component, **yoga** combines mindful breathing with poses that improve strength and flexibility. Though known for its calm, flow-like sequences, yoga can be adapted to any fitness level, ensuring it is accessible to people of all ages and abilities. Practitioners often report lower cortisol levels, elevated mood, and improved cardiovascular markers after regular practice.

Families can adopt short, playful yoga sessions at home, transforming them into bonding activities. Young adults juggling school or job pressures can schedule brief "yoga breaks" to centre themselves before diving back into hectic schedules. In either scenario, mindful movement fosters a balanced intersection of body, breath, and mental focus.

Integrating Mindfulness into Daily Routines

- **Morning Check In**: Spend 2–3 minutes practising breath awareness as soon as you wake up.

- **Mindful Eating**: During meals, chew slowly, savour flavours, and notice texture and aroma—rather than rushing.

- **Midday Reset**: Pause for a brief body scan, especially if tension creeps into your neck or back.

- **Pre-Bed Wind-Down**: Guided meditations can help transition from a busy day to a restful state, promoting deeper, more refreshing sleep.

By consistently weaving mindfulness into your day, you develop greater emotional resilience. Over time, you will notice heightened clarity, reduced anxiety, and a host of benefits for your heart, including steadier blood pressure and healthier resting heart rates.

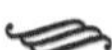

Relaxation Techniques for Emotional and Physical Relief

Progressive Muscle Relaxation

While mindfulness addresses stress at its cognitive root, **progressive muscle relaxation** focuses on dissolving physical tension. The method is straightforward:

1. **Choose a Quiet Space**: Lie comfortably, close your eyes, and take a few slow, deep breaths.

2. **Tense and Release**: Begin with your toes, tensing them firmly for about 5 seconds. Exhale and release. Progress upward through your

calves, thighs, torso, arms, and neck, pausing to feel the wave of relaxation after each release.

3.   **Observe Sensations**: Tune into the difference between tension and relaxation. This process builds your awareness of bodily stress signals.

Performing a full-body scan in this way can offer instant relief. Over time, it sharpens your ability to self-regulate muscular tension, mitigating stress's adverse effects on heart rate and blood pressure.

Visualisation: Crafting a Mental Retreat

Visualisation involves creating vivid mental images of peaceful scenarios, such as a sunlit beach, a tranquil mountain lake, or a secret garden. By immersing yourself in these serene landscapes—focusing on sights, sounds, smells, and textures—you effectively redirect your mind from daily hassles to a safe haven of calm. Physiologically, visualisation can slow breathing and reduce tension in the body, which translates to fewer stress-induced fluctuations in heart function.

Practical Tip: If you find it challenging to conjure visual scenes, pair visualisation with calming music or nature sounds. This multisensory experience can deepen the therapeutic effect, making sustaining a tranquil mental state easier.

Aromatherapy and Calming Music

For centuries, diverse cultures have harnessed scents to influence mood and promote relaxation. **Aromatherapy** uses essential oils—like lavender, chamomile, and bergamot—to evoke calm, reduce anxiety, and support emotional wellness. Diffuse your chosen oil in the background while doing daily tasks, add a few drops to a warm bath, or keep an essential oil roller bottle handy for quick application to pulse points.

Soothing music can similarly modulate stress responses. Slow-tempo tracks or nature-based sounds (e.g., rainfall, ocean waves, bird songs) have been linked to lower heart rates and reduced anxiety. In fact, any genre that personally resonates—classical, ambient, light jazz—can serve as a potent emotional balm, transporting your thoughts away from tension and into a more harmonious mental space.

Combining Relaxation Strategies

While each relaxation technique works well, combining them can amplify their benefits. Imagine pairing progressive muscle relaxation with aromatherapy: as you tense and release your muscles, the gentle scent of lavender nurtures an even more profound release of tension. Or visualise a tranquil forest scene while listening to instrumental music softly playing in the background. Engaging multiple senses anchors you in relaxation, helping you disconnect from external stressors.

Building Consistency: The true power of relaxation strategies emerges when they become part of your everyday routine. By practising them regularly—rather than waiting until you are overwhelmed—your body learns to recover from stress more quickly. Over time, these moments of calm accumulate, fostering a resilient mental and cardiovascular state.

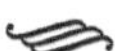

Creating a Stress-Free Environment

Decluttering for Clarity

Our surroundings subtly influence our mood and stress levels. A cluttered desk, an overflowing laundry basket, or a chaotic living area can signal to the mind that life is disorganised. That sense of disarray can spark anxiety and impede relaxation. According to Rohanshah (2023), organised environments often reduce stress and enhance productivity.

Practical Tip: Begin the decluttering journey incrementally—tackle one shelf, drawer, or area at a time. Assign categories like "keep," "donate," or "discard." A single clean corner of a room can spur motivation to continue organising.

Minimalist Design and Natural Elements

Once you have decluttered, you might explore **minimalist design** principles, emphasising simplicity and function. Clear surfaces and intentional décor can generate an air of calm, reflecting your intention to keep stress at bay. Research from Schahaff (2024) links minimalist living arrangements to improved mood and creativity.

Bringing **nature indoors**—with houseplants, natural light, or nature-inspired art—has been shown to reduce stress by up to 15% and elevate mood by about 25%. For families, creating a cosy nook near a window where sunlight streams in can foster shared moments of relaxation. For young adults in smaller living spaces, a single plant or a sunlit desk space can infuse a sense of calm.

Personal Comforts and Tech-Free Zones

Personalising your space can help you form an emotional attachment that encourages serenity. Family photos, cherished travel souvenirs, or mementos with meaningful backstories transform your environment into a tapestry of positive memories. These personalised touches serve as visual reminders that evoke joy and tranquillity.

Equally crucial is setting up **tech-free zones**—areas where screens are prohibited. Chronic digital engagement can heighten stress, disrupt sleep, and undermine face-to-face interactions. By designating device-free spaces, you nurture mindful living, deeper relationships, and calmer energy within the home.

1. **Dining Spaces**: Keep smartphones off the table, focusing instead on conversation and mindful eating.

2. **Reading Nooks**: Reserve a corner of your living room or bedroom as a sanctuary for reading physical books or journaling.

3. **Bedrooms**: Encourage better sleep by avoiding screens at least 30 minutes before bedtime.

Sustaining a Serene Environment

Maintaining a calm, organised home or workspace is an ongoing process rather than a one-time event:

- **Regular Check-Ins**: Schedule monthly mini-reviews of clutter. Donate items you no longer use and tidy areas that may have slipped back into disarray.

- **Family Collaborations**: Involve children or partners by assigning each person a small part of the home to organise. This fosters teamwork and consistent upkeep.

- **Positive Reinforcement**: Celebrate the improvements—however small—and take a moment to acknowledge how these adjustments make you feel more relaxed and in control.

You create a supportive backdrop for mindful living and heart health by carefully shaping your physical environment. Each decluttered surface, cosy corner, or patch of sunlight contributes to a home that actively counters stress rather than amplifies it.

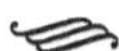

Developing Healthy Coping Mechanisms

Physical Activity and Heart Health

When stress mounts, it is tempting to slip into unhealthy coping patterns—like overeating, isolating oneself, or relying on screens for distraction. In contrast, **regular physical activity** offers a constructive channel for releasing stress-induced energy and tension. Exercise stimulates the production of endorphins, and your body's natural mood enhancers, simultaneously lowering levels of stress hormones like cortisol.

- **Aerobic Activities**: Walking, jogging, or swimming can sharpen mental clarity, help regulate blood pressure and strengthen cardiac function.

- **Strength Training**: Lifting weights or doing bodyweight exercises supports muscular health and boosts confidence and emotional well-being.

- **Family Fitness**: Families can plan weekend hikes, bike rides, or dance sessions, seamlessly combining social bonding with heart-healthy habits.

Creative Outlets

Human beings are inherently creative; harnessing this creativity can yield a profound sense of purpose and stress relief. **Artistic pursuits**—such as painting, music, writing, or sculpting—serve as conduits for emotional expression. Rather than bottling up frustration or worry, you can channel these feelings into colours on canvas or notes in a song.

Group Engagement: Young adults or families could organise craft nights or creative workshops. Group art projects foster collaboration, empathy, and collective joy, all of which combat isolation, a common by-product of chronic stress.

Social Support Networks

No one is meant to navigate life entirely alone. **Quality relationships** can buffer against stress, offering reassurance, guidance, and laughter during challenging times. Whether it is a friend who listens without judgement or a mentorship group that resonates with your passions, investing time in building these relationships can significantly lower stress levels.

- **Shared Activities**: Joining clubs, church groups, or volunteer organisations can expand your community and introduce you to diverse individuals who can broaden your support system.

- **Family Dinners**: Regular shared meals encourage open communication, allowing each member to discuss daily challenges and victories.

- **Peer Support**: Young adults entering new jobs or college can benefit from campus organizations, hobby clubs, or even digital communities that align with their interests.

Balanced Nutrition for Emotional Resilience

An often overlooked factor in stress management is **diet**. Nutrient-dense foods—rich in vitamins, minerals, and antioxidants—fortify your body against stress's physical toll. They also help stabilise blood sugar and energy levels, making emotional regulation easier.

- **Whole Foods**: Fruits, vegetables, lean proteins, and whole grains provide vital nutrients that fuel both body and mind.

- **Omega-3 Fatty Acids**: Found in fish (e.g., salmon, mackerel), walnuts, and flaxseeds, omega-3s support brain health and can reduce inflammation linked to stress responses.

- **Probiotics and Prebiotics**: A healthy gut microbiome influences mood and hormone balance. To nourish beneficial gut bacteria, include yogurt, kefir, kimchi, or high-fibre fruits.

Family meal planning, cooking sessions, or potluck-style gatherings encourage positive eating habits and create an environment where balanced nutrition becomes the norm.

Integrating Coping Skills into Everyday Life

1. **Plan & Set Goals**: Clearly define how to incorporate exercise, creative pursuits, or social engagements into your weekly schedule.

2. **Experiment & Adapt**: Try cycling or dancing if you find daily walks boring. If painting feels forced, explore writing or photography. Variety keeps coping mechanisms fresh and enjoyable.

3. **Celebrate Small Wins**: Completing a 20-minute workout, finishing a short journal entry, or preparing a healthy meal is worthy of acknowledgement. Each small success propels you closer to a heart-healthy lifestyle.

By proactively selecting positive outlets for stress, you transform negative tension into personal growth, emotional resilience, and improved cardiovascular health.

Final Thoughts

Mastering stress management is about more than addressing fleeting moments of anxiety; it is a holistic commitment that reverberates through every facet of your life—especially your heart health. From identifying subtle daily irritations to implementing structured coping strategies, stress management fosters a resilient mind and body.

Here is a Recap of Key Strategies:

1. **Identify Sources of Stress**

   - Use journaling and self-assessment tools to reveal hidden triggers.

- Lean on supportive friends, family, or professionals for insights and guidance.

2. **Practice Mindfulness and Meditation**

- Adopt breath awareness, guided meditations, or body scans to ground yourself.

- Incorporate mindful movement, such as yoga, to unify physical and mental relaxation.

3. **Harness Relaxation Techniques**

- Experiment with progressive muscle relaxation, visualisation, aromatherapy, and soothing music.

- Combine methods for a richer, multisensory approach to stress relief.

4. **Create a Stress-Free Environment**

- Declutter living spaces and integrate minimalist, nature-infused design elements.

- Personalise your surroundings with meaningful objects and establish tech-free zones.

5. **Develop Healthy Coping Mechanisms**

- Engage in physical activity to release tension and strengthen heart health.

- Explore creativity—through art, music, or writing—to channel emotions productively.

- Cultivate strong social connections and adopt balanced nutrition to support emotional equilibrium.

These insights are especially valuable for families aiming to build a supportive household and young adults preparing for long-term wellness. By implementing these tools, you safeguard your cardiovascular health and elevate your day-to-day life, gaining clarity, emotional stability, and a renewed sense of control.

Remember: Stress is not a signal of personal failure; it is an inherent part of living in a demanding world. Proactively recognising its sources, learning healthier responses, and refining your environment to minimise triggers all protect your heart. Whether you are a busy parent juggling responsibilities or a student navigating new challenges, the techniques outlined in this chapter can guide you towards a life of greater serenity and robust well-being.

Embrace each method step by step, remain patient with yourself, and understand that true mastery of stress takes consistent effort and time. Gradually, you will discover that the power to manage stress and support your heart health rests in your own hands—and that realisation alone can be an immense source of peace.

Power of Restorative Sleep

Sleep is not a luxury but a foundational pillar that sustains physical and mental health. This chapter explores the profound connection between sleep and heart health, detailing how insufficient or poor-quality rest can significantly raise the risk of cardiovascular problems. You will learn about the different stages of sleep and their impact on heart function, discover how hormonal balance and inflammation levels are influenced by nightly rest, and identify the ramifications of chronic sleep deprivation. In addition, we will discuss establishing an effective bedtime routine, recognising common sleep disorders, optimising your bedroom environment for deeper rest, and integrating daily activities that support consistent, restorative sleep. By the end, you will understand why prioritising high-quality slumber can transform your heart and overall well-being.

Understanding the Sleep-Heart Connection

The goal of the Subpoint

Highlight the intrinsic link between sleep and cardiovascular function, emphasising how each stage of the sleep cycle, along with hormonal regulation and inflammation control, plays a vital role in heart health.

Sleep Stages and Heart Function

Why Sleep Stages Matter

When we drift off each night, our brains, and bodies cycle through distinct phases of sleep that collectively form what researchers call "sleep architecture." These stages include light sleep (N1), deeper slow-wave sleep (N3), and rapid eye movement (REM) sleep. Each has a critical impact on bodily recovery, emotional regulation, and cardiovascular health.

1. **Stage N1 (Light Sleep)**: This is the transitional stage where you move from wakefulness to sleep. Though brief, it sets the tone for the rest of the night. During this period, your heart rate starts to slow, shifting the body into restorative modes.

2. **Stage N2:** Your heart rate and breathing become more regular, and body temperature drops. This phase usually occupies the largest chunk of total sleep time, reinforcing the stabilisation of physiological functions.

3. **Stage N3 (Deep/Slow-Wave Sleep):** Here, brain waves slow down significantly, and the body goes into intense repair mode. In this phase, the heart gets a rare opportunity to operate at a reduced rate, lowering blood pressure and promoting beneficial changes for cardiovascular tissues.

4. **REM Sleep:** Named for the rapid eye movements observed in this stage, REM sleep is associated with dreaming, memory consolidation, and emotional processing. Heart rate can fluctuate during REM, but overall, it helps integrate stress-coping mechanisms and emotional resilience, indirectly supporting cardiovascular health.

When these stages flow seamlessly, your heart benefits from periodic rest, reduced blood pressure, and improved heart rate variability (HRV). Research in multiple cardiology journals (Huang, T. et al.) has shown that HRV often increases in individuals with regular, uninterrupted sleep cycles, indicating a heart that adapts well to changes in rest and activity.

Heart Rate Variability and Cardiovascular Health

Heart rate variability (HRV) is the fluctuation in time intervals between each heartbeat. A higher HRV suggests that your autonomic nervous system (ANS) – which controls functions like heart rate, digestion, and respiratory rate – is flexible and well-regulated. When you achieve prolonged deep sleep and robust REM cycles, the parasympathetic ("rest-and-digest") branch of your ANS gains a foothold, leading to better HRV. Conversely, fragmented sleep can suppress parasympathetic activity, elevating stress hormones and increasing risk factors for cardiovascular ailments like hypertension and arrhythmias.

Consequences of Sleep Disruptions

Recurring arousals from noise, the environment, or underlying sleep disorders can curtail the total time spent in deep sleep (N3) and REM. These disturbances lead to higher nighttime cortisol levels, hinder the gradual dip in blood pressure known as "nocturnal dipping," and result in greater cardiovascular strain over time. According to the American Heart Association, individuals who consistently experience these disruptions are more susceptible to heart attacks, heart failure, and other vascular complications.

Hormonal Regulation during Sleep

Stress Hormones and Heart Function

Cortisol, a key stress hormone, naturally peaks in the early morning to help you wake up and gradually declines throughout the day. Nighttime cortisol levels drop during healthy sleep, allowing your heart rate and blood pressure to settle. However, if your sleep is fragmented or too short, cortisol may remain excessively high, undermining the recuperative benefits that your heart seeks at night.

Additionally, the hormone epinephrine (adrenaline) can surge in response to poor sleep, creating a state of chronic sympathetic overactivity. This scenario forces your cardiovascular system to operate in near-constant stress mode, escalating the likelihood of plaque formation in the arteries and elevating the risk of stroke.

Insulin and Cortisol Balance

Insulin—a hormone vital for regulating blood sugar—also depends on consistent, high-quality sleep for proper functioning. Insufficient sleep lowers insulin sensitivity, prompting the body to compensate for producing more insulin. Over time, this insulin resistance can pave the way for metabolic disorders like type 2 diabetes, which further jeopardise heart health.

When you fail to rest enough, cortisol's antagonistic role against insulin can intensify. Elevated cortisol levels disrupt glucose metabolism, ramp up appetite, and often lead to poor dietary choices, placing an even heavier burden on the heart. This cyclical dynamic—reduced sleep leading to hormonal imbalances and subsequent cardiovascular stress—is why many heart disease prevention programmes underscore the necessity of better rest alongside diet and exercise.

Sleep and Inflammation

Inflammatory Markers and Cardiac Risk

Inflammation serves as the immune system's natural reaction to injuries or infections. However, chronic low-grade inflammation can damage arterial walls and accelerate plaque accumulation, creating an environment ripe for heart attacks and strokes. Quality sleep is a nightly "reset button," helping the body clear inflammatory by-products and regulate immune responses. Studies cited by the Centers for Disease Control and Prevention reveal that even a few nights of insufficient sleep can elevate levels of inflammatory markers like C-reactive protein (CRP).

Sleep Deprivation as an Inflammatory Trigger

When the body never fully enters or sustains slow-wave sleep, the immune system remains in a semi-alert state, producing more cytokines that perpetuate inflammation. As a result, crucial cardiovascular tissues endure steady wear, contributing to hardening or narrowing of arteries (atherosclerosis). Chronic inflammation also aggravates other risk factors such as high cholesterol, high blood pressure, and obesity, weaving a complex web that puts the heart at continual risk.

Long-term Sleep Deprivation Effects

Elevated Risks for Heart Conditions

Long-standing sleep debt—regularly clocking fewer than 6 hours per night— has been linked to a wide spectrum of cardiovascular issues, from coronary artery disease to arrhythmias. NIH Research Matters confirms that irregular and inadequate sleep can produce a profound negative impact on long-term heart health.

Habitual Poor Sleep and Hypertension

Blood pressure naturally dips during deeper sleep stages. If your nights are punctuated by awakenings or shortened rest, your body can't achieve this beneficial "dip." Over time, consistently higher nocturnal blood pressure translates to greater daytime blood pressure, increasing the strain on vessel walls and amplifying the risk of strokes or congestive heart failure.

Sleep Deprivation: A Modifiable Risk Factor

While age, genetics, and environmental stressors can be challenging to control, improving your sleep is an initiative-taking step you can take. Setting regular bedtimes, improving your sleep environment, and seeking help for persistent issues transform sleep from a health vulnerability into a robust protective factor. Recognising chronic tiredness as a modifiable contributor to heart disease underscores the urgency of making deeper, longer, and more consistent sleep a priority.

Establishing a Bedtime Routine

Goal of the Subpoint

To provide concrete, actionable steps for creating an evening routine that facilitates better rest, directly reinforcing cardiovascular health.

Consistent Sleep Schedule

Why Bedtimes and Wake up Times Matter

Your body's internal clock, or circadian rhythm, relies heavily on consistency. Fluctuating bedtimes disrupt the synchronisation of hormones, including melatonin and cortisol, which are central to managing sleep-wake cycles. Adhering to a fixed bedtime and wake-up time—even on weekends—"trains" your brain to recognise when it is time to wind down and when to perk up.

Tailoring to Your Lifestyle

If your job requires early mornings, aligning your bedtime accordingly is vital to consistently get the recommended 7–9 hours of sleep. Conversely, night shift workers may need specialised schedules and light-management strategies (like blackout curtains) to establish a reversed, but still consistent, routine. Families, especially those with children, can benefit from communal wind-down rituals, promoting an environment where everyone respects and values regular rest.

Relaxation Techniques Before Bed

Reading, Deep Breathing, and Meditation

A pre-sleep routine with calming activities helps transition your body from a stimulated "fight-or-flight" mode to a more relaxed, parasympathetic state. This can include:

- **Reading**: Choose calming, non-work-related material such as fiction or uplifting non-fiction to distract your mind from daily pressures.

- **Deep Breathing**: Techniques like box breathing (inhale for 4 seconds, hold for 4, exhale for 4, and hold again for 4) slow heart rate and reduce muscle tension.

- **Meditation**: Guided mindfulness apps or 5–15 minutes of silent meditation can clear anxious thoughts, resetting your emotional state before lights out.

Relaxation practices benefit your heart by dialling down adrenaline levels and stabilising heart rate. Over time, you will notice you fall asleep faster, experience fewer nighttime awakenings, and wake up feeling more refreshed.

Limiting Screen Time

Blue Light and Melatonin Suppression

Electronic devices emit light that mimics daylight to our brain, making it challenging to produce sufficient melatonin (the hormone that cues us for bedtime). Excessive evening screen exposure—whether from a phone, tablet, computer, or TV—delays the onset of crucial sleep stages.

Strategies to Curb Overstimulation

- **Tech Curfew**: Set a hard cutoff, such as no screens after 9:00 pm. This boundary helps reduce late-night scrolling or streaming binges.

- **Night Mode**: Many devices include "night shift" or "blue light filter" options that reduce blue light emission. Though helpful, these filters are not a substitute for powering down entirely.

- **Screen-Free Zone**: Keep all electronics out of the bedroom. Opt for a standalone alarm clock rather than your smartphone if an alarm is necessary.

Creating a Sleep-Inducing Environment

The Value of a Pre-Bed Sanctuary

A tranquil bedroom sets the stage for uninterrupted sleep, essential for the heart's nightly recovery. Your bed should symbolise rest and comfort—avoid using it as a workspace, TV lounge, or dining area if possible.

Personal Rituals that Reinforce Rest

Simple rituals can shape your bedroom into a sanctuary: lightly spritzing lavender essential oil on pillows, dimming lamps 30 minutes before bedtime, or playing calming music. Over time, these cues inform your brain that it is time to transition into rest, aligning your psychological state with the body's circadian rhythms.

The Impact of Sleep Disorders

Goal of the Subpoint

To shed light on common sleep disorders—insomnia, sleep apnoea, and others—explaining how each condition poses substantial risks to heart health and when to seek professional help.

Overview of Common Sleep Disorders

Insomnia, Sleep Apnoea, Restless Leg Syndrome, and More

While occasional sleep disruptions happen to everyone, persistent issues may indicate an underlying sleep disorder. Among the most frequent are:

- **Insomnia**: Characterised by ongoing difficulty falling or staying asleep. Often linked with stress, anxiety, or irregular schedules.
- **Obstructive Sleep Apnoea (OSA)**: Periodic breathing pauses due to airway blockages, causing brief awakenings and oxygen deprivation.

- **Restless Leg Syndrome (RLS):** Uncomfortable leg sensations trigger an urge to move them, commonly preventing seamless transitions into deeper sleep.

- **Narcolepsy:** Less common but involves sudden sleep attacks and difficulty regulating normal sleep-wake cycles.

Recognising these disorders is critical for heart health, as untreated cases frequently contribute to high blood pressure, inflammation, and metabolic issues over time.

Sleep Apnoea and Heart Health

Mechanics of Sleep Apnoea

In obstructive sleep apnoea, relaxation of throat muscles narrows air passages, causing breathing pauses. Sleep cycles are disturbed each time your body jolts you awake to resume airflow. This repeated stress on the cardiovascular system can raise nighttime blood pressure, which often carries over into the daytime.

Managing Sleep Apnoea

Treatments include lifestyle modifications – weight loss, reducing alcohol intake, adjusting sleep positions – and medical interventions like CPAP (Continuous Positive Airway Pressure) machines that keep airways open. Specialised dental appliances or surgical options may also be considered. Early identification is paramount; the longer sleep apnoea remains undiagnosed, the greater the cumulative strain on your heart.

Insomnia and Stress Impact

Physiological Consequences

Chronic insomnia involves prolonged sleep latency (taking too long to fall asleep) or difficulties staying asleep throughout the night. This condition can keep the sympathetic nervous system persistently active, elevating heart rate and blood pressure. Over months or years, these cardiovascular burdens can heighten your vulnerability to atherosclerosis or other heart conditions.

Therapeutic Approaches

Cognitive Behavioural Therapy for Insomnia (CBT-I) remains the gold standard for addressing insomnia's root causes. By reframing negative thought patterns about sleep, you can lessen anxiety and stress, thereby reintroducing healthier sleep cycles. Relaxation strategies and good sleep hygiene further reinforce the health benefits of consistently deep rest.

Seeking Professional Help

Why Timely Intervention Matters

Sleep disorders rarely disappear on their own and can progress from mild to severe. Prolonged lack of proper treatment allows damaging cycles—involving cortisol spikes, metabolic dysregulation, and inflammatory responses—to intensify. This can raise the risk of heart attacks, strokes, or chronic heart failure.

Diagnostic and Treatment Pathways

If you suspect a sleep disorder, begin with a healthcare professional or a sleep specialist. Options such as overnight polysomnography (sleep study), home sleep apnoea tests, or mental health evaluations can clarify the underlying issues. Armed with an accurate diagnosis, medical teams can recommend personalised solutions, whether that is a CPAP device for apnoea, sleep medication for short-term insomnia, or comprehensive therapy for chronic RLS.

Improving Sleep Quality through Environment

Goal of the Subpoint

Offer tangible methods to transform your sleeping space into a peaceful retreat, thereby maximising the body's ability to engage in deep restorative sleep and protect heart health.

Optimising Bedroom Darkness

Melatonin and Sleep Onset

Melatonin is integral to signalling the body that it is time to wind-down. Even low light sources—like a glowing bedside clock or LED indicators from electronics—can confuse your biological clock. According to the Sleep Foundation, ensuring near-complete darkness helps preserve higher melatonin levels, supporting easier sleep onset.

Practical Darkness Solutions

- **Blackout Curtains**: Ideal for blocking external lights, especially for shift workers.

- **Eye Masks**: A budget-friendly alternative if modifying the room is not feasible.

- **Dimming or Covering Electronics**: Place a small cover over the bright LED on your modem or switch off devices entirely.

Controlling Noise Levels

Noise Pollutants and Their Effects

Subtle noises might seem harmless, but repeated disruptions can jolt you out of deep sleep, reducing overall sleep efficiency. Chronic exposure to nighttime noise—like passing traffic or even a partner's snoring—prevents the cardiovascular system from fully relaxing. Over time, this can escalate stress hormone production and increase heart strain.

Practical Noise Control

- **White Noise or Sound Machines**: A steady ambient sound can camouflage sudden noises.

- **Earplugs**: Inexpensive yet effective for many, blocking intermittent disruptions.

- **Strategic Furniture or Soundproofing**: Plush furniture, rugs, or acoustic panels in the bedroom can dampen external noise, shielding you from jarring awakenings.

Setting Comfortable Temperature

Thermoregulation and Sleep Cycles

Your core body temperature naturally dips in preparation for rest. If your bedroom is too warm—above 70°F (21°C)—it can interrupt this thermoregulatory process. Cooling the room encourages your body to slip into deeper sleep more quickly.

Tips for an Optimal Climate

- **Thermostat Adjustments**: Aim for a bedroom temperature between 60–67°F (15–19°C).

- **Bedding Choices**: Lightweight, breathable materials can keep you cool in hotter climates, whereas heavier duvets or blankets may be suitable in colder regions.

- **Fans and Air Circulation**: Good airflow helps dispel heat and humidity, preventing you from overheating at night.

Ergonomic Bedding Choices

Supporting Spinal Alignment

If you consistently wake up with aches, your mattress or pillow may be underperforming. Proper spinal alignment—where the neck, spine, and hips align neutrally—can reduce nocturnal fidgeting, enhance deep sleep, and help maintain a stable heart rate.

Finding the Right Bedding

- **Mattress Type**: Memory foam, latex, or hybrid mattresses offer varying degrees of firmness. Prioritise comfort and support.

- **Pillow Height and Firmness**: Back sleepers need thinner pillows to keep the neck aligned, while side sleepers do better with thicker, firmer pillows.

- **High-Quality Sheets**: Natural fibres like cotton or bamboo can wick moisture and regulate body temperature, easing the burden on the heart by promoting deeper rest.

Balancing Sleep and Daily Activities

Goal of the Subpoint

Explain how daily habits—from exercise timing to dietary choices—can be optimised to support better nighttime rest, reinforcing the cardiovascular system's ability to recover and rejuvenate.

Establishing a Daily Routine

Why Structure Matters

Random daily schedules can wreak havoc on your circadian rhythm. By creating predictability—regular times for meals, work, exercise, and relaxation—you help your body modulate energy levels more efficiently. This stability translates to a smoother transition into sleep, improving the heart's capacity for overnight repair.

Sample Daily Framework

- **Morning**: Rise at a consistent time, expose yourself to bright light (sunlight or a light therapy box), and have a balanced breakfast.

- **Midday**: Include a moderate physical activity break, such as a short walk or low-intensity workout.

- **Late Afternoon**: Wind-down from high-intensity tasks; reduce caffeine intake to avoid nighttime restlessness.

- **Evening**: Prepare a lighter dinner, limit screen use before bed, and engage in calming wind-down routines (e.g., reading or light stretching).

Mindful Scheduling of Exercise

Timing Is Key

Exercise is a well-known ally for heart health: it improves cardiac efficiency, regulates blood pressure, and supports weight management. Yet timing your workouts strategically can optimise your sleep. High-intensity sessions too late in the day elevate core body temperature and adrenaline levels, making it tough to settle into sleep. Aim for vigorous workouts earlier, leaving gentler routines (like yoga or leisurely walks) for the evening.

Exercise Benefits for Sleep

Regular exercisers often experience shorter sleep onset latency and more substantial time in slow-wave sleep. A brisk walk in the morning or a moderate workout mid-afternoon can help stabilise mood and reduce stress, easing the mental load that often hampers nighttime relaxation. By reinforcing the body's natural inclinations towards movement and rest, you sustain healthy circadian rhythms that favour heart recuperation.

Dietary Considerations

Heavy Meals and Sleep Quality

Digestion can disrupt comfort if a meal is eaten too close to bedtime—particularly if it is fatty, spicy, or high in sugar. Late-night eating can also trigger acid reflux, forcing you to wake up multiple times. A heavy meal can drive your body into a prolonged digestion phase rather than channelling energy toward restorative processes.

Caffeine and Alcohol

Caffeine has a half-life of around 5–6 hours, meaning an afternoon cup of coffee could remain in your system at bedtime. Try limiting caffeine intake to mornings or early afternoons to avoid sleep disturbances. Similarly, although alcohol may induce initial drowsiness, it disrupts deeper REM stages later, creating fragmented sleep and heightening cardiac stress.

Implementing Wind-Down Activities

Smooth Transition to Slumber

The final 30–60 minutes of the day set the stage for how well you will rest. Engaging in relaxing practices—writing in a gratitude journal, listening to soothing music, or indulging in mild stretching—helps the mind detach from daily hassles and the heart shift into a lower gear.

Examples of Wind-Down Routines

- **Gentle Yoga**: Simple poses (like Child's Pose or Legs-Up-the-Wall) calm the nervous system.

- **Aromatherapy**: Scents like lavender or chamomile can encourage tranquillity.

- **Light Reading or Mindful Colouring**: Engaging in calming tasks that do not involve bright screens.

Key Takeaways

1. **Sleep is Essential for Heart Health**

   Each sleep stage—especially deeper slow-wave and REM phases—contributes to cardiovascular repair and stress relief.

2. **Consistent Routines Strengthen Cardiac Recovery**

   Maintaining regular bedtimes, relaxation rituals, and screen-free zones foster deeper sleep cycles, which better support heart function.

3. **Sleep Disorders Demand Attention**

   Conditions like sleep apnoea, insomnia, or restless leg syndrome can dangerously raise blood pressure and inflammation. Early intervention is paramount.

4. **Optimising Your Environment Pays Off**

   Darkness, comfortable temperatures, noise control, and ergonomic bedding collectively shape a haven for healthy sleep.

5. **Daily Habits make a difference**

   Thoughtful exercise scheduling, balanced meal timings, and wind-down activities all enhance the benefits of a full night's rest.

Conclusion

Your heart tirelessly beats day in and day out, but it relies on consistent, high-quality sleep to replenish and maintain optimal function. From regulating hormones and reducing inflammation to providing the downtime necessary for tissue repair, a full night's rest is a core component of sustaining cardiovascular health. By establishing bedtime routines, addressing potential sleep disorders, enhancing your sleeping environment, and managing your daily activities wisely, you can significantly bolster your heart's resilience. Whether you are a busy parent, a professional juggling deadlines, or someone eager to maximise well-being, making restorative sleep a priority is one of the most impactful choices you can make for your heart and your life.

The Love Prescription:
Social Support for a Stronger Heart

The Love Prescription delves into the close link between social connections and heart health, highlighting how meaningful relationships can powerfully influence our cardiovascular well-being. While many focus on diet and exercise to protect their hearts, this chapter underscores an equally critical factor: our social ties. Introducing the idea of love as a "prescription" for a stronger heart prompts readers to reflect on the types of connections they cultivate every day.

Readers will learn how supportive social ties function as a vital safeguard against cardiovascular disease, as well as an essential component in managing it. The chapter offers scientific evidence illustrating how nurturing relationships can ease stress and fortify heart function by releasing beneficial hormones like oxytocin. In discussing several types of social support—emotional, instrumental, and informational—it draws on relatable examples, whether aimed at families wanting to improve collective health or young adults exploring new fitness routines. This focus on social nuances provides valuable insight into creating networks that foster community, shared responsibility, and better heart health for all.

Introduction to the Love Prescription

In a quiet suburb, an elderly man named Harold had been living alone since the passing of his beloved wife. His isolation weighed heavily on him, both emotionally and physically, as evident in rising blood pressure levels and growing concerns about his cardiovascular well-being. Then one day, his neighbour Mary noticed his solitude and began to visit him regularly. Over cups of tea and conversations about their gardens, Harold discovered a renewed sense of purpose. His spirits lifted, and to his surprise, his heart health indicators improved at his next check-up. While he had changed neither his diet nor his exercise routine, these positive shifts were attributed to the genuine human connection rekindled by Mary's caring presence.

Harold's experience illustrates the importance of quality over mere proximity when it comes to social support. Meaningful relationships do more than offer company; they provide emotional relief that can tangibly boost physical health. A strong sense of being loved and supported lowers stress, which in turn benefits the heart through reduced blood pressure and healthier heart rate variability.

In this chapter, "love" is not limited to romance. Instead, it covers the broader realm of emotional, social, and psychological support. It represents a listening ear in tough times, a reassuring hug after a difficult day, or the gentle encouragement that helps us overcome life's hurdles. These comforting ties function as anchors, providing stability during life's storms and fuelling emotional resilience.

Although the idea of social support as a form of medical intervention may seem unconventional, research backs up its significance. Much like doctors prescribe medications for heart conditions, one could envision prescribing "love" as part of a holistic heart health plan. In many ways, love counteracts stress, lessens inflammation, and enhances circulation. When we "prescribe love," we focus on creating environments rich in uplifting relationships, ensuring individuals feel supported and less burdened by life's demands.

Understanding how these relationships protect heart health requires looking at the body's physiological responses. In supportive social settings, the body releases oxytocin, often called the "love hormone." This hormone calms the cardiovascular system by offsetting stress-inducing hormones such as cortisol and adrenaline. Through positive, loving interactions, we harness these powerful biological processes to guard the heart.

Because we can control how we build and maintain our social ties, strengthening relationships becomes a compelling way to protect ourselves from cardiovascular disease. It is a vital reminder that self-care should go beyond counting calories or miles on the treadmill; it should also include forging and maintaining meaningful bonds with others. For families aiming for better collective health, planning group walks, sharing home-cooked meals, or volunteering together can reinforce both social and cardiovascular wellness. Young adults likewise benefit from dedicating time to friendships and community involvement, enriching their lives while bolstering their hearts against stress.

Focusing on social support enriches conventional heart health approaches with elements of empathy and mutual care. By acknowledging how love and friendship contribute to well-being, readers are encouraged to seek out and nurture positive connections. Incorporating these relationships into everyday life transforms the path to sustained heart health into a communal effort—reminding us that we are not alone in pursuing better well-being.

The idea of a "love prescription" urges readers to treat their social networks as invaluable contributors to heart health. Simple yet powerful actions—reaching out to a lonely neighbour, joining local groups, or setting aside quality time for loved ones—bring us closer to stronger hearts. Embracing this mindset not only enhances personal health but also builds communities grounded in compassion and understanding.

Scientific Foundations of Social Support and Heart Health

The dynamic interplay between social support and cardiovascular health has intrigued scientists for decades. Early research found that people with strong social connections often have lower rates of heart disease, revealing a critical link between emotional well-being and physical health. These initial discoveries set the stage for further investigation into how our bonds with others affect us biologically.

Over time, studies revealed that stress hormones such as cortisol and adrenaline significantly influence heart health. When under stress, the body releases these hormones, leading to elevated blood pressure, a faster heart rate, and inflammation—all potential risk factors for heart disease. Persistent stress due to weak or nonexistent social networks compounds these risks, placing loneliness on par with well-known risk factors like smoking or obesity.

Conversely, positive social experiences stimulate the release of oxytocin, the "love hormone." Oxytocin soothes stress responses and lowers inflammation, playing a pivotal role in nurturing a healthy cardiovascular system. Regular exposure to this hormone supports heart function and aids in recovery following cardiac events. For example, multiple studies, including one in the *Journal of the American College of Cardiology*, highlight better outcomes and quicker recovery times for heart attack patients who enjoy strong social support.

By reducing blood pressure and heart rate through supportive interactions, social ties encourage a sense of safety and belonging. Over time, these factors can contribute significantly to cardiovascular resilience. Moreover, beneficial social contact lessens inflammation – a key factor in heart disease progression – through the release of anti-inflammatory compounds during positive, meaningful engagement.

Importantly, the benefits hinge on the quality rather than the sheer number of connections. One or 2 deeply supportive relationships can be far more protective for heart health than a large network lacking genuine closeness. This distinction underscores that it is not quantity, but rather the consistency, positivity, and true backing of relationships that matter most.

Diverse Forms of Social Support

Social support comes in different forms, each with its significance for heart health. **Emotional support** involves empathy, caring for words, and attentive listening. These gestures help relieve emotional strain and buffer against chronic stress, directly safeguarding cardiovascular well-being. Families that practice compassion and validation within their homes find it easier to make and stick to collective heart-healthy decisions.

Instrumental support centres on practical help—providing transport to doctor's appointments, sharing homemade meals, or assisting with household tasks. Such tangible aid can be vital for managing everyday challenges and preventing stress overload, thereby promoting a healthier heart. For young adults juggling multiple responsibilities, a well-organised support network enables them to dedicate more attention to exercise, healthy meal preparation, and stress management.

Informational support addresses the need for knowledge, offering credible advice or resources on maintaining a healthy heart. Whether via digital forums, library materials, or local community initiatives, reliable information about nutrition, exercise, and mental health helps people make informed choices. Being part of an online group that discusses heart-healthy recipes or shares exercise tips can motivate sustained progress and foster a sense of belonging.

However, not all forms of support are automatically helpful. **Healthy support** respects boundaries and empowers independence, while **unhealthy support**—such as excessive interference or controlling behaviour—can create stress and hinder personal growth. Overbearing assistance leads to reliance or resentment, while constructive guidance preserves everyone's autonomy.

To maintain beneficial dynamics, clear communication and active listening are crucial. For instance, when providing emotional support, genuinely tuning in to another person's feelings and acknowledging their concerns reinforces trust. In terms of instrumental support, scheduling specific times to lend a hand can prevent misunderstandings or overwhelm. When offering information, ensuring resources are evidence-based and relevant safeguards against misinformation and confusion.

Regularly revisiting and adjusting support methods is also essential. Families could set up routine check-ins to discuss how well current arrangements are working, while young adults might rely on fitness apps or online communities to gauge progress and stay connected. Over time, consistent, well-balanced support fosters a supportive environment that prioritises heart health for everyone involved.

Relationships and Their Impact on Heart Health

Romantic partnerships have a direct influence on cardiovascular health. Partners who embrace joint goals—such as nutritious cooking at home or taking daily walks together—create strong routines that reinforce each other's well-being. Conversely, tension or ongoing disagreements may escalate stress levels, increasing blood pressure and stress hormone production. Consequently, healthy communication and shared objectives in a relationship become essential safeguards for heart health.

For **families**, generational habits and customs can shape heart health positively or negatively. Certain cultural diets, like the Mediterranean pattern, focused on fresh produce and healthy fats, can foster robust cardiovascular function. Other inherited eating practices, however, might amplify risk factors if high in salt, sugar, or unhealthy fats. Ensuring clear discussions around health expectations and boundaries can help align family members towards heart-friendly habits.

Friends also play a pivotal role, whether through emotional support or influence on lifestyle. Sharing health goals with peers often encourages positive behaviours, such as group workouts or social gatherings centred on nutritious meals. Still, be mindful that certain social circles could normalise habits detrimental to the heart, such as smoking or binge drinking.

Additionally, **pets and community groups** expand our support networks. The companionship of animals can ease loneliness and promote regular physical movement, such as walking a dog. Community organisations, charities, or faith-based groups provide shared purpose, emotional solace, and practical help, cultivating a wider circle of support that benefits heart health.

In all these relationships, striking a balance is vital. Couples can strengthen their bond and health by setting mutual targets, families can relieve tensions with open communication, and friends should encourage constructive habits. By recognising and managing potential stressors, relationships stay consistently supportive rather than becoming burdensome.

Practical Applications and Challenges

To harness the power of social support, begin by **evaluating your current network**. Pinpoint individuals who offer different types of support—emotional, practical, or informational—and see where gaps exist. Someone would love to help more if they realised the need. Charting out this network clarifies existing resources and highlights areas for improvement.

Next, **strengthen emotional connections** through open, regular communication. Discuss anxieties, celebrate milestones, and explore mutual activities that promote both physical and emotional health. Cooking together, attending exercise classes, or volunteering as a group fosters deeper connections while advancing shared wellness goals.

When offering or receiving support, **maintaining boundaries** is essential to prevent burnout. Caregivers should be honest about their limitations to avoid overwhelm, and those accepting help should respect and appreciate these boundaries. By clearly laying out expectations, support systems remain beneficial and manageable for everyone involved.

Leveraging **technology** can make the process more structured. From smartphone apps tracking daily steps or heart rate to online forums connecting people with similar health goals, digital tools expand the reach of social support. Forming an "accountability partnership" with someone committed to consistent check-ins further enhances motivation and ensures continuity of effort.

Bringing It All Together

Throughout this chapter, we have seen how social connections function as a foundational pillar for preventing and managing heart disease. The story of Harold and Mary exemplified how a simple, genuine effort to be present can spark transformative improvements in heart health. In examining scientific evidence, we learned how positive interactions release oxytocin, reduce harmful stress hormones, and strengthen the cardiovascular system. This perspective shifts the conversation about heart health from a narrow focus on diet and exercise to a more comprehensive view that includes the vital impact of relationships.

Families and young adults alike can cultivate these supportive bonds by prioritising empathy, open communication, and communal activities. By placing as much importance on companionship as on other health measures, individuals take active steps towards a holistically healthier lifestyle. Ultimately, recognising the power of love, friendship, and community in shaping heart health encourages us to integrate social ties into our daily wellness routines. In doing so, we affirm that the pursuit of a strong heart is truly a shared journey—one that is enriched by the connections we value and nurture along the way.

Set Your Heart Free: The Transformative Power of Avoiding Risky Substances

Introduction

A healthy heart is not simply the result of a single choice or action. Instead, it reflects the sum of many daily decisions, from how we move our bodies and what we put on our plates, to how we cope with stress. Each of these elements contributes to the vitality of our cardiovascular system and our overall well-being. Among these factors, avoiding risky substances stands out as particularly crucial. Whether it is tobacco, excessive alcohol, or recreational drugs, these substances pose a significant threat to heart health.

In fact, within the 6 pillars of lifestyle medicine, "avoidance of risky substances" is regarded as the most direct measure to protect the heart. This chapter explores why these substances are so damaging, offers guidance on how to reduce or eliminate them, and highlights how these changes can transform not just your cardiovascular health but every facet of your life.

Knowledge is Power—but Action is Essential

It is often said that knowledge is power, and learning about the risks posed by harmful substances is an important first step. Recognising the impact these substances have on arteries, blood pressure, and heart function can spark the desire to change. Yet, knowledge alone rarely ensures success. Quitting or avoiding tobacco, excessive alcohol, or other harmful substances often requires a solid plan, steadfast support, and abundant patience. People commonly make multiple attempts before a new habit finally sticks—and that is entirely normal.

Our goal in this chapter is twofold: to provide information about how substances like tobacco and alcohol affect cardiovascular health, and to inspire hope. We'll discuss strategies for coping with cravings, handling peer pressure, and replacing harmful habits with healthier ones. We'll also look at how lifestyle medicine incorporates other vital components—such as regular physical activity, a balanced diet, effective stress management, and sufficient sleep—to nurture the heart as comprehensively as possible.

The Power of Consistency and Self-Compassion

A healthy heart thrives on consistency, self-compassion, and the determination to keep trying. Breaking free from risky substances can be one of life's biggest challenges, yet it is also one of the most liberating. Positive changes to the cardiovascular system begin surprisingly soon after that final cigarette or once you cut back on alcohol. Within days, you can move towards lower blood pressure, better circulation, and improved cholesterol profiles. Over months and years, these benefits grow exponentially, sharply reducing your risk of heart disease, heart failure, and stroke.

Think of this chapter as your guided resource where you can learn about harmful substances, understand how they endanger your heart, and find clarity on the way forward. Whether you are reading for yourself or a loved one, remember that you have the power to make healthier choices. While the journey towards a substance-free lifestyle may be challenging, it is a path well worth taking. Through patience and support, you can not only avoid risky substances but also thrive in their absence, unlocking a more vibrant and heart-healthy life.

Why "Avoidance of Risky Substances" Matters

Lifestyle medicine rests on 6 foundational pillars: nutrition, physical activity, stress management, sleep, social connections, and avoidance of risky substances. Together, these pillars form a resilient framework for long-term health. At its core, the pillar of "avoidance of risky substances" recognises that certain substances—when used habitually or excessively—undermine heart health. Tobacco (including cigarettes, cigars, or e-cigarettes), excessive alcohol, and various recreational drugs all threaten the cardiovascular system.

Avoiding these substances can be the most direct way to safeguard heart health. While the other pillars focus on risk factors like obesity, stress, and poor nutrition, this pillar addresses the fundamental question of what you put into your body. For those already living with heart disease or with elevated risks—like high blood pressure or high cholesterol—avoiding risky substances becomes even more critical. Tobacco, heavy alcohol use, and stimulants like cocaine can significantly increase the chances of heart attack, stroke, or heart failure.

Yet, breaking free from these substances is often one of the toughest behavioural changes to undertake. Nicotine is famously addictive, making cigarettes or e-cigarettes intertwined with daily routines and social habits. Alcohol, similarly, can become a go-to for celebrations or stress relief, complicating efforts to cut back. And recreational drugs present their own set of complexities, such as psychological dependence and mental health issues. Despite these hurdles, the rewards can be profound: people who succeed in avoiding or stopping substance use often see swift improvements in heart function and enjoy the broader health benefits that follow.

The Tobacco Trap: Why Smoking Spells Trouble for Your Heart

Tobacco use remains one of the most significant contributors to heart disease worldwide. Although smoking rates have declined in some regions, it still ranks as a major cause of preventable deaths.

How Tobacco Damages the Heart

When you inhale cigarette smoke, you introduce over 7,000 chemicals into your lungs. Hundreds of these are toxic, and around 70 are known carcinogens. Nicotine is a powerful vasoconstrictor that narrows blood vessels, raising blood pressure and forcing the heart to work harder. Over time, this strain increases the risk of chest pain (angina), abnormal heart rhythms (arrhythmias), and eventually heart failure.

Smoking also damages the lining of the arteries, paving the way for plaque buildup (atherosclerosis). This restricts blood flow and is a key factor in developing coronary artery disease, peripheral artery disease, and cerebrovascular disease (which can lead to stroke). Even secondhand smoke poses risks to anyone who inhales it, underscoring the dangers for both smokers and those around them.

Quitting: The Sooner, the Better

The good news is that quitting smoking can reverse many of these effects surprisingly quickly. Research shows that the risk of cardiovascular problems starts to drop within a day of quitting. After a year, a former smoker's heart disease risk can fall to about half that of a current smoker. With continued abstinence, the risk eventually nears that of a person who has never smoked at all. The body's ability to repair damaged blood vessel linings and restore normal function is remarkable, provided the toxic chemicals are no longer present.

However, quitting smoking is rarely straightforward. Many people try multiple times before they succeed. Nicotine replacement therapies (patches, gum, or lozenges), prescription medications, behaviour modification programmes, and support from friends, family, or quit lines can all help. Every cigarette not smoked is a small but important triumph for your heart.

The Ripple Effect of Quitting Tobacco

Giving up tobacco offers more than just heart health benefits. It lowers your risk of various cancers, improves lung function, and can save you a substantial amount of money. Psychologically, overcoming addiction can boost self-esteem and a sense of personal power. From a purely cardiovascular standpoint, however, avoiding tobacco is one of the most effective ways to add healthy years to your life.

Alcohol: Where Is the Line Between Moderate and Excessive?

Alcohol differs from tobacco in that some research suggests moderate consumption—up to one drink a day for women and up to 2 for men—may offer certain cardiovascular benefits, such as a slightly lower risk of coronary artery disease. However, these findings are hotly debated, and individual factors like genetics, diet, and lifestyle can complicate the picture.

The Risks of Heavy Drinking

What is clear is that heavy drinking poses a serious threat to heart health. Binge drinking or regularly exceeding recommended guidelines can heighten the risks of heart attack, heart failure, stroke, and high blood pressure. Over time, copious amounts of alcohol can weaken the heart muscle (alcoholic cardiomyopathy) and trigger arrhythmias like atrial fibrillation, which increases the risk of stroke if unmanaged.

High-calorie alcoholic beverages can also contribute to weight gain, which in turn raises the risk of elevated blood pressure, unhealthy cholesterol levels, and type 2 diabetes. Additionally, those with pre-existing heart conditions should be especially cautious, as alcohol can exacerbate existing problems.

Finding Balance

If you choose to drink, many experts recommend spreading out your intake across 3 or more days per week instead of consuming several drinks in a single sitting. This approach eases the strain on your cardiovascular system and helps prevent binge drinking. Some individuals—such as those with liver disease, a history of addiction, or adverse medication interactions—should avoid alcohol entirely.

What constitutes a "safe" amount of alcohol varies from person to person. Factors like age, body mass, genetics, and underlying health conditions all play a role. If you are uncertain whether alcohol is safe for you, consult your healthcare provider. They can help you determine whether any potential heart benefits outweigh the risks in your unique case.

Beyond Tobacco and Alcohol: Other Risky Substances

While tobacco and alcohol receive the most attention, a variety of recreational and illicit drugs also endanger heart health. Stimulants like cocaine, methamphetamine, and misused prescription medications can raise blood pressure and cause irregular heartbeats. Opioid misuse introduces additional dangers, including respiratory depression that can indirectly affect heart function.

Cocaine and Stimulants

Cocaine is infamous for causing acute cardiovascular problems—such as heart attacks and arrhythmias—even in young people with no prior heart issues. Its powerful vasoconstrictive effect makes the heartbeat faster and blood vessels tighten, creating enormous strain. Chronic use increases the risk of atherosclerosis, meaning even occasional "party" use can have lasting consequences.

Opioids and Other Depressants

Opioids primarily slow down the respiratory system, reducing oxygen flow to vital organs. In the event of an overdose, a lack of oxygen can lead to heart damage, brain damage, or death. While opioids do not always seem as directly hazardous to the heart as stimulants, their overall toll on the body can be severe, especially when they are mixed with other substances.

Marijuana and Emerging Substances

Marijuana use raises heart rate and blood pressure for short periods, and any form of smoking can irritate the cardiovascular and respiratory systems. Synthetic cannabinoids (like "Spice" or "K2") may cause unpredictable cardiovascular effects, from mild heartbeat elevation to severe arrhythmias.

Any substance that strains the heart, disrupts normal blood pressure or heartbeat, or encourages plaque buildup can be deemed risky. Quitting or minimising these substances promotes better heart health and safeguards other organs vulnerable to substance-related harm.

Overcoming Addictions: Patience, Support, and Steps to Success

The Nature of Addiction

Addiction occurs when certain behaviours—often related to substance use—become compulsive, even as they cause harm. It is driven by changes in brain chemistry, emotional triggers, and entrenched habits. Addiction is not a moral failing but a chronic condition that typically requires long-term management, support, and resilience. Recognising that relapse is common in recovery can help maintain perspective and momentum.

Stages of Change

Healthcare professionals often reference the Transtheoretical Model (Stages of Change) to understand how people break free from addictive behaviours:

1. **Precontemplation:** The individual is not considering quitting or is unaware of the problem.

2. **Contemplation:** Awareness of the problem grows, though ambivalence may persist.

3. **Preparation:** The person intends to act soon and starts gathering resources or setting a quit date.

4. **Action:** Tangible steps are taken—disposing of substances, entering rehab, or starting medication.

5. **Maintenance:** The person focuses on preventing relapse by building healthier habits and coping skills.

6. **Relapse (Potential):** A return to old behaviours, which can offer lessons to refine future strategies.

Each stage calls for different interventions and support systems. A relapse does not erase previous progress; it can highlight areas that need attention.

Practical Strategies for Quitting

1. **Set Clear Goals:** Define what quitting means to you. It is a firm quit date for tobacco or a plan to gradually reduce alcohol intake. Clear, realistic goals create a roadmap for change.

2. **Seek Professional Help:** Healthcare providers, counsellors, and addiction specialists can offer personalised treatment plans, including nicotine replacement therapy or prescription medications, and cognitive behavioural therapy (CBT) for various addictions.

3. **Build a Support Network:** Friends, family, support groups (like Alcoholics Anonymous or SMART Recovery), or online forums can provide invaluable encouragement and accountability. Sharing your experiences can make all the difference.

4. **Identify Triggers:** Learn to recognise the people, places, emotions, or times of day that provoke cravings. Developing strategies to handle these triggers—like going for a walk instead of smoking or meditating instead of pouring a drink—can help replace harmful patterns.

5. **Consider Replacement Habits:** Rather than simply removing a substance from your life, replace it with healthy activities. Exercise, new hobbies, or relaxation techniques like deep breathing can ease the sense of loss and reinforce your substance-free path.

6. **Track and Celebrate Progress:** Use a journal, app, or milestone announcements to mark each victory. Small achievements—like a week without cigarettes or a month without binge drinking—help you see how far you have come and motivate you to continue.

The Role of Patience and Support

Recovery from substance use is rarely linear. Expect twists, turns, triumphs, and setbacks. Patience—from both yourself and those around you—is crucial. Societal stigma can create additional barriers, but compassion and understanding are far more effective in guiding someone to lasting change. If you are a loved one supporting someone in recovery, offer encouragement without judgement. If you are the one breaking free, practice self-care, accept the possibility of relapse, and view each new day as a chance to strengthen your resolve.

Closing Thoughts

Avoiding risky substances is an essential pillar in the quest for a healthy heart. While overcoming addiction or changing long-standing habits can feel daunting, the benefits for your cardiovascular system—and your overall health—are well worth the effort. By pairing determination with compassionate support, you can free your body and mind from the grip of harmful substances, opening the door to a more vibrant, heart-healthy life.

Harnessing the Power of Supplements

Maintaining a healthy heart requires a balanced approach that includes a nutritious diet, regular exercise, stress management, and sufficient sleep. Yet even the most devoted individuals may struggle to get all the nutrients necessary for peak cardiovascular function through diet alone. This is where supplements can play a pivotal role. By filling nutritional gaps and supporting heart health in targeted ways, certain supplements can help improve cholesterol levels, reduce inflammation, and enhance overall cardiovascular well-being. In this chapter, we'll delve into the key supplements that can fortify your heart health, explain how they work, and offer practical tips for integrating them into your daily routine.

Understanding the Role of Supplements

Supplements are not meant to replace a healthy lifestyle; rather, they are designed to complement nutritious eating habits, consistent exercise, and effective stress management. Because the heart works around the clock—pumping oxygen and nutrients throughout the body—it needs a steady supply of specific vitamins, minerals, and fatty acids to maintain its resilience.

- **Improve Cholesterol Profiles:** Many supplements help raise HDL (the "good" cholesterol) while lowering LDL (the "bad" cholesterol).

- **Reduce Inflammation:** Chronic inflammation is a primary risk factor for heart disease, and certain nutrients have proven anti-inflammatory effects.

- **Enhance Blood Vessel Function:** Better vascular health leads to improved blood flow and lower blood pressure.

- **Protect Against Oxidative Stress:** Antioxidant-rich supplements can help guard cells and blood vessels against oxidative damage that accelerates plaque formation.

Below, we examine the most significant supplements for heart health and highlight the scientific evidence that supports their benefits.

1. Omega-3 Fatty Acids

Why They Matter:

Omega-3 fatty acids, found in fatty fish like salmon and mackerel, are some of the most thoroughly studied supplements for cardiovascular health. They are considered essential fats because the body cannot produce them independently and must obtain them from dietary or supplemental sources.

How They Work:

- Lower triglycerides and reduce harmful inflammation.
- Help regulate healthy heart rhythms.
- Aid in preventing arterial plaque buildup.
- Contribute to the production of prostaglandins, hormone-like substances that support overall cardiovascular function.

Recommended Dose:

Aim for 1,000–2,000 mg per day of combined EPA (eicosapentaenoic acid) and DHA (docosahexaenoic acid). These are typically available in fish oil capsules or algae-based supplements for those following a vegetarian or vegan diet.

Tips for Use:

- Choose third-party-tested products to avoid contaminants such as mercury.
- Take omega-3s with meals to enhance absorption and minimise any fishy aftertaste.

Food for Thought:

If you eat fatty fish at least twice a week, you might already be meeting your omega-3 needs. However, supplementation can be helpful for individuals who dislike fish or have dietary restrictions.

2. Coenzyme Q10 (CoQ10)

Why It Matters:

CoQ10 is a naturally occurring antioxidant found in every cell in the body. It plays a crucial role in mitochondrial energy production and is particularly important for heart health because the heart muscle has exceptionally high energy demands.

How It Works:

- Supports the creation of ATP, the energy molecule essential for cellular functions.

- Acts as an antioxidant, reducing oxidative stress and preventing the oxidation of LDL cholesterol – a crucial factor in plaque development.

- Levels naturally decline as we age, and certain medications (notably statins) can deplete CoQ10.

Recommended Dose:

100–300 mg per day.

Tips for Use:

- Ubiquinol (the active form of CoQ10) is more readily absorbed than ubiquinone. Opt for ubiquinol if you are over 40 or concerned about absorption.

- Take CoQ10 with a meal containing healthy fats to improve its uptake by the body.

Food for Thought:

If you are on statins, CoQ10 supplementation becomes even more critical to help counteract the medication's tendency to lower natural CoQ10 levels.

3. Magnesium

Why It Matters:

Magnesium is involved in over 300 biochemical reactions within the body, many of which are directly tied to cardiovascular health. Despite this, magnesium deficiency is surprisingly common, partly due to depleted soils and modern food processing methods.

How It Works:

- Relaxes blood vessels, thereby helping to lower blood pressure.

- Supports a consistent heartbeat and helps regulate muscle contractions, preventing spasms in the heart and blood vessels.

- Plays an essential role in energy metabolism and nerve function.

Recommended Dose:

300–400 mg per day.

Tips for Use:

- Forms such as magnesium citrate or glycinate are well absorbed and gentler on the stomach.

- Dividing the total daily dose into 2 or 3 smaller doses can minimise gastrointestinal issues.

Food for Thought:

Although dark leafy greens, nuts, seeds, and whole grains are great sources of magnesium, many people still do not get enough from their diets, making supplementation a wise option.

4. Fibre Supplements

Why It Matters:

Fibre is a key player in controlling cholesterol levels and maintaining overall heart health. A diet rich in fibre is also associated with better weight management and more stable blood sugar levels.

How It Works:

- Soluble fibre binds to cholesterol in the gut, preventing it from being absorbed into the bloodstream.

- Encourages healthy digestion and helps control appetite, which can lead to better weight and cardiovascular outcomes.

- Reduces spikes in blood sugar, a principal factor in reducing the risk of heart disease.

Recommended Dose:

Aim for a total of 25–30 grams of fibre per day, with 5–10 grams coming from soluble fibre.

Tips for Use:

- Psyllium husk is a well-researched fibre supplement known to be effective in lowering LDL cholesterol.

- Increase fibre intake gradually and drink plenty of fluids to prevent digestive discomfort.

Food for Thought:

Fibre supplements work best alongside a high-fibre diet rich in fruits, vegetables, beans, and whole grains, creating a synergistic effect for heart protection.

5. Vitamin D

Why It Matters:

Nicknamed the "sunshine vitamin," vitamin D has a multitude of roles in the body, including immune support and hormone regulation. Its impact on heart health is increasingly recognised, particularly concerning blood pressure regulation and arterial function.

How It Works:

- Regulates calcium in the bloodstream, helping maintain flexible, healthy arteries.

- Alleviates inflammation, a significant contributor to cardiovascular disease.

- Low levels of vitamin D are linked to an increased likelihood of hypertension, heart attacks and strokes.

Recommended Dose:

1,000–4,000 IU daily, depending on your blood levels, latitude, and the amount of sunlight you receive.

Tips for Use:

- Regular blood tests are the best way to determine if you are deficient.

- Combining vitamin D with vitamin K2 helps ensure that calcium goes into your bones rather than your arteries.

Food for Thought:

While your body can produce vitamin D through skin exposure to sunlight, factors like geography, climate, and lifestyle can limit your ability to synthesise enough naturally.

6. L-Carnitine

Why It Matters:

L-carnitine is an amino acid derivative vital for energy production, particularly in the heart, which relies heavily on fatty acids for fuel.

How It Works:

- Transports fatty acids into the cell's mitochondria, where they are burned for energy.

- Enhances blood flow and may reduce symptoms associated with angina and heart failure by improving energy metabolism in the heart muscle.

Recommended Dose:

1-3 grams daily, split into 2 or 3 doses.

Tips for Use:

- Taking L-carnitine alongside CoQ10 can provide additional benefits for cellular energy.

- Acetyl-L-carnitine offers added cognitive support if you are also interested in brain health.

Food for Thought:

While red meat is a natural source of L-carnitine, relying on excessive amounts of red meat could have drawbacks, making supplementation a more consistent way to achieve therapeutic levels.

7. Garlic Extract

Why It Matters:

Garlic is famous in the culinary world, but its benefits extend beyond flavour. Research shows that it supports cardiovascular health through several mechanisms, such as lowering cholesterol and blood pressure.

How It Works:

- Allicin, the active compound in garlic, helps relax blood vessels and reduce inflammation.

- Garlic can modestly lower LDL cholesterol levels and offer mild antiplatelet activity, which lowers the likelihood of blood clots.

Recommended Dose:

600–1,200 mg of aged garlic extract daily.

Tips for Use:

- Aged garlic extract tends to be odourless and contains concentrated amounts of beneficial compounds.
- Use in tandem with a balanced, heart-healthy diet for optimal results.

Food for Thought:

Although raw garlic can be potent, it is challenging to maintain a consistent allicin dose through diet alone, making supplements a practical alternative.

8. Antioxidants: Vitamin E and Selenium

Why They Matter:

Oxidative stress speeds up the development of heart disease by damaging blood vessels and accelerating plaque buildup. Antioxidants like vitamin E and selenium help counteract these harmful processes.

How They Work:

- Vitamin E protects LDL cholesterol from oxidative damage.
- Selenium is crucial to produce glutathione, a major antioxidant in the body that helps neutralise free radicals.

Recommended Dose:

- Vitamin E: 15 mg daily.
- Selenium: 55–100 mcg daily.

Tips for Use:

- Look for natural (d-alpha-tocopherol) forms of vitamin E for better bioavailability.
- Avoid high-dose antioxidant supplementation unless specifically advised, as too much can be counterproductive.

Food for Thought:

Brazil nuts are an excellent source of selenium; eating just one per day can often provide your entire daily requirement.

9. Plant Sterols and Stanols

Why They Matter:

Plant sterols and stanols naturally resemble cholesterol in their structure, enabling them to effectively decrease cholesterol absorption in the intestines.

How They Work:

- Compete with dietary cholesterol, leading to lower LDL levels in the bloodstream.
- Reduce the overall risk of plaque accumulation in arteries.

Recommended Dose:

2–3 grams daily.

Tips for Use:

- Many functional foods, such as certain margarines and orange juices, are fortified with plant sterols and stanols.
- Combine them with regular exercise and a balanced diet for a more robust cholesterol-lowering strategy.

Food for Thought:

Pairing plant sterols with soluble fibre can yield a powerful one-two punch for reducing LDL cholesterol.

10. Resveratrol

Why It Matters:

Resveratrol is a polyphenol found in red wine, grapes, and certain berries. It has generated interest in its anti-inflammatory and heart-protective qualities.

How It Works:

- Improves endothelial function by helping blood vessels dilate more effectively.

- Offers antioxidant properties that mitigate oxidative stress and mild antiplatelet benefits.

Recommended Dose:

100–200 mg daily.

Tips for Use:

- Supplements are a more reliable source than relying on red wine for resveratrol intake, especially for those who avoid alcohol.

- Products that combine resveratrol with other polyphenols can provide enhanced synergy.

Food for Thought:

Grapes, blueberries, and cranberries naturally contain resveratrol, so adding these foods to your diet can support heart health in conjunction with supplementation.

The Art of Supplementing Safely

While supplements can offer notable advantages, approaching them thoughtfully is crucial:

1. **Consult Your Doctor**

   Always talk to a healthcare provider before introducing new supplements, particularly if you are taking medications or have existing health concerns.

2. **Start Slowly**

   Add only one supplement at a time. This method allows you to track its effects and watch for any adverse reactions.

3. **Choose Quality**

4. Opt for reputable brands that practise third-party testing. This ensures purity, potency, and safety.

If you have specific questions or need personalised guidance, feel free to contact **Dr Jitesh Arora** at drjitesharora@gmail.com.

Integrating Supplements Into a Heart-Healthy Lifestyle

Even the best supplements cannot replace the foundational elements of heart health. To achieve the greatest impact, combine your chosen supplements with:

- **A Nutritious Diet**

  Focus on whole, unprocessed foods, including fruits, vegetables, whole grains, legumes, and lean proteins.

- **Regular Physical Activity**

  Exercise strengthens the heart and helps maintain optimal circulation.

- **Stress Management**

  Techniques such as meditation, yoga, deep breathing, or journaling can reduce the chronic stress that harms cardiovascular function.

By adopting a well-rounded strategy—supplements included—you offer your heart the comprehensive support it deserves, allowing it to continue beating strongly for years to come.

Key Takeaway

When used wisely and in tandem with a healthy lifestyle, supplements serve as valuable allies in your quest for a robust cardiovascular system. They help bridge nutritional gaps, minimise inflammation, lower cholesterol, and protect against oxidative damage—all of which contribute to a healthier, more resilient heart.

Heartfelt Transformations: Real Journeys with Lifestyle Medicine

In recent years, using lifestyle medicine to prevent, treat, and even reverse chronic diseases has gained remarkable traction. From diet and exercise to stress management and social connections, simple daily habits can work wonders—especially for heart health. This chapter shares the real-life stories (composites inspired by actual cases) of 5 Indo-American patients, aged 28 to 60, who dramatically improved their heart health by integrating the 6 pillars of lifestyle medicine: nutrition, physical activity, stress management, sleep, avoiding harmful substances, and social bonds. Each person's journey highlights the powerful impact of intentional lifestyle changes in creating lasting well-being.

1. Aarav Patel, 35: Overcoming Early Hypertension

Background

At 35, Aarav Patel had a successful tech career. As a father of 2 and the main breadwinner, his frantic schedule left little time for self-care. Frequent headaches, constant fatigue, and occasional dizziness prompted a visit to the doctor, where he was diagnosed with Stage 1 hypertension – an early warning sign that his cardiovascular system was under strain.

Journey with Lifestyle Medicine

1. **Nutrition**

   Aarav's daily fare mirrored a typical American diet: fast-food lunches, regular restaurant dinners, and sugary snacks to beat the afternoon slump. Acting on his doctor's advice, he embraced a plant-focused diet. Drawing on his Indian heritage, he created healthier versions of beloved dishes like dal, sabzi, and roti by reducing oil and salt. He switched from white rice to brown rice and quinoa, replacing soda with lime-infused water or herbal tea. These small but consistent shifts drastically cut his intake of sodium and sugar.

2. **Physical Activity**

    Making time for exercise in his 10-hour workday was challenging, so Aarav introduced 2 short, 15-minute walks during breaks and a 30-minute evening workout. He cycled on a stationary bike while catching up on emails some nights. On weekends, he played soccer with friends or took his kids to the park, turning physical activity into valuable family time.

3. **Stress Management**

    Juggling professional demands, parenting, and extended family obligations made Aarav anxious. He started with 5 minutes of deep breathing each morning before the rest of the household woke up, gradually adding guided meditation apps. Over time, his stress levels fell, and he noticed he was calmer at work.

4. **Sleep**

    Aarav previously survived on 5 or 6 hours of restless sleep. Determined to do better, he set a strict bedtime, limited screen time in the evenings, and dimmed the lights to help his body wind-down. Soon he slept a steady 7 hours each night, with more energy in the mornings and less dependence on caffeine.

5. **Avoiding Harmful Substances**

    Although Aarav enjoyed social drinks on weekends and at office gatherings, he chose to limit himself to a single glass of wine or a light beer, eventually trying alcohol-free options. He quickly realised he could still be social without overindulging.

6. **Social Bonds and Connections**

    Aarav enlisted the support of his family, sharing his new health objectives. His parents began cooking lighter meals for family get-togethers, his wife joined him for evening walks, and his coworkers encouraged his daily breaks. This circle of support fortified his commitment and kept him motivated.

Outcome

Within 6 months, Aarav's blood pressure stabilised. He was 10 pounds lighter at a follow-up visit, and his blood work was markedly better. His doctor applauded the changes. By adjusting his diet, prioritising exercise, and managing stress effectively, Aarav controlled his hypertension without medication—while reclaiming precious time and energy for his family.

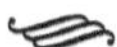

2. Shilpa Sharma, 44: Triumph Over High Cholesterol

Background

Shilpa Sharma, a 44-year-old entrepreneur, believed she was "too young" to worry about heart disease—until a routine test showed alarmingly high cholesterol levels. With a family history of early heart disease, she knew she needed a radical shift. At the helm of a demanding start-up, Shilpa routinely worked 16-hour days, fuelled by caffeine and fast-food takeout.

Journey with Lifestyle Medicine

1. **Nutrition**

   Alarmed by her lipid panel results, Shilpa met with a registered dietitian who recommended a fibre-rich meal plan. She phased out fried snacks in favour of roasted chickpeas, almonds, and fruit. Rather than relying on takeout, she used meal prep services once weekly, ensuring she had portioned, home-cooked meals. This helped reduce her intake of saturated fats while increasing whole grains, fruits, and vegetables.

2. **Physical Activity**

   Shilpa had always hated treadmills, so her coach suggested dance-based workouts and yoga. She discovered a nearby Bollywood dance fitness class that not only honoured her cultural roots but also helped her work up a sweat in a fun, social environment. She looked forward to dancing 3 times a week and found genuine joy in movement.

3. **Stress Management**

   The intense pressures of launching and running a start-up often left Shilpa stressed. She began taking brief "breathing breaks" throughout the day, stepping away from her screen to do quick breathing exercises or stretches. She also started a nightly journal, listing 3 things she was grateful for, which helped reframe her thoughts and calm her mind before bed.

4. Sleep

Shilpa realised her chronic stress was robbing her of restorative sleep. In response, she created a "wind-down" routine: a warm shower, turning down the lights, and turning off electronic devices 30 minutes before bedtime. The improvement in her sleep was immediate—she began waking up refreshed, no longer feeling the usual morning fog.

5. Avoiding Harmful Substances

Overwhelmed by her workload, Shilpa occasionally relied on smoking to cope. Determined to make lasting changes, she sought counselling to quit. Gradually, she replaced the urge to smoke with deep breathing or herbal teas, noticing improvements in both taste and smell, and a surge in overall energy.

6. Social Bonds and Connections

Friends and family rallied behind her, offering support, and even joining her Bollywood fitness classes. They exchanged healthy recipes and shared daily motivational texts that kept Shilpa accountable and encouraged her to keep going.

Outcome

After 3 months of consistent effort, Shilpa saw a marked improvement in her cholesterol. Her LDL ("bad") cholesterol dropped by 25 points, while her HDL ("good") cholesterol rose. She felt more energised, less bogged down by stress, and more confident in growing her start-up—knowing she was protecting her heart for the future.

3. Nikhil Singh, 60: Reclaiming Life After a Cardiac Event

Background

Sixty-year-old Nikhil Singh experienced a mild heart attack while visiting family in India. That harrowing event reminded him that he needed to change his habits. Upon returning home to the United States, he reflected on his long-held routines—lengthy workdays as an accountant and social gatherings rich in fatty foods and sweets—that had contributed to his condition.

Journey with Lifestyle Medicine

1. **Nutrition**

    Under the guidance of a cardiologist and a nutritionist, Nikhil was introduced to a heart-healthy diet focused on fruits, vegetables, whole grains, and lean proteins like fish and legumes. Adapting his much-loved Indian recipes meant trimming down on ghee and full-fat cream, relying more on aromatic spices—cumin, turmeric, coriander—to boost flavour without unhealthy fats.

2. **Physical Activity**

    Following his heart attack, Nikhil enrolled in a cardiac rehabilitation programme that offered supervised exercise sessions. He started slowly, walking on a treadmill and pedalling a stationary bike, gradually increasing speed and resistance. After rehab, he joined a local gym, where he added light weights to his routine. His physical strength and endurance improved, as did his sense of well-being.

3. **Stress Management**

    Coming face-to-face with mortality pushed Nikhil towards better stress management. He explored meditation and pranayama (yogic breathing techniques) and rediscovered the peacefulness he had not realised he was missing. Engaging in gardening also helped him relax, combining physical activity with a meditative, outdoor hobby.

4. **Sleep**

    Late-night TV and social media scrolling had previously taken a toll on Nikhil's sleep. Post-heart attack, he committed to 7 or 8 hours of quality rest. Cutting back on evening screen time and adopting a more relaxed bedtime ritual that included reading and deep breathing made an enormous difference in both the quantity and quality of his sleep.

5. **Avoiding Harmful Substances**

   Nikhil was not a heavy smoker but indulged occasionally at social events. After his cardiac scare, he quit smoking entirely—no exceptions. His once-regular glass of whisky or beer at gatherings became an occasional treat, often replaced with non-alcoholic drinks or fruit-infused water.

6. **Social Bonds and Connections**

   Support from loved ones played a critical role in his recovery. His wife prepared heart-healthy dishes, and they began taking evening walks together. His adult children called regularly to check in and cheer him on. Feeling surrounded by concern and encouragement, Nikhil remained motivated to keep his heart in top shape.

Outcome

A year after his heart attack, Nikhil felt stronger than he had in years. His cardiologist noted significant improvements in his cardiovascular tests, blood pressure, and cholesterol. By focusing on better nutrition, regular exercise, and effective stress management, Nikhil not only fortified his heart but also rediscovered a deep appreciation for life.

4. Ria Iyer, 50: Beating Prediabetes and Heart Risk

Background

At 50, Ria Iyer found herself balancing her career as a community college educator with caring for her ageing parents. She was gaining weight around her midsection, constantly tired, and craving sugar. Tests confirmed prediabetes and elevated triglycerides, both of which indicated a heightened risk for heart disease.

Journey with Lifestyle Medicine

1. **Nutrition**

    Raised on homemade Indian sweets and carb-heavy curries, Ria realised she needed to adapt her diet. Working with a certified diabetes educator, she cut back on refined carbs and bulked up on non-starchy vegetables. She swapped white rice for cauliflower rice and moong dal to stabilise her blood sugar and added protein (like Greek yogurt, tofu, or lentils) to keep her energy levels even.

2. **Physical Activity**

    With her packed schedule, Ria found it tough to get to the gym, so she took brisk walks around campus after lunch. She also discovered online yoga classes and began practising in the early mornings. By focusing on consistency rather than intensity, she managed to integrate these new habits into her busy life.

3. **Stress Management**

    Tending to her job and her parents often left Ria stressed. She started a simple gratitude ritual, recording 3 positive moments each day. She also listened to soothing music or podcasts during her commute. Gradually, her stress levels declined, and she felt more in control of her mood and appetite.

4. **Sleep**

    Late-night grading sessions and Netflix binges had previously disrupted Ria's rest. Determined to prioritise sleep, she organised her work more efficiently—grading papers earlier and delegating some household tasks—to stick to a consistent bedtime. As a result, she regularly got 8 hours of quality sleep, improving both her energy and focus.

5. **Avoiding Harmful Substances**

    Ria did not smoke, but she was partial to several cups of sweet, milky chai each day. She reduced the sugar in her tea, sometimes adding cinnamon for a hint of sweetness. This small shift cut her daily sugar intake significantly and helped stabilise her blood glucose levels.

6. **Social Bonds and Connections**

    Ria›s siblings and extended family helped care for her parents, giving her some much-needed relief. She also joined a local support group for caregivers, where she found advice and solidarity. Sharing experiences encouraged her to keep prioritising her own health.

Outcome

After 6 months, Ria's blood work showed that her prediabetes had reversed, and her triglycerides dropped into a healthier range. By restructuring her diet, staying active, and managing stress and sleep, she not only avoided a looming diabetes diagnosis but also rediscovered energy for both work and family.

5. Samar Roy, 31: Conquering Obesity and Heart Risk

Background

Thirty-one-year-old Samar Roy faced a strong family history of type 2 diabetes and heart disease. Working long hours in the hospitality sector, he frequently reached for high-calorie meals—pizza, pastries, and sugary iced coffee. Troubled by breathlessness even on short stair climbs and borderline high blood pressure, Samar knew he needed to act before his cardiovascular risks became a reality.

Journey with Lifestyle Medicine

1. **Nutrition**

    Determined to make a change, Samar began controlling his portions, filling half his plate with vegetables and the other half with lean protein and whole grains. He replaced the vending machine snacks with nuts, seeds, and fruit. Using a food-tracking app helped him spot hidden sugars and cut unnecessary calories. Gradually, he felt more satisfied on fewer calories.

2. **Physical Activity**

Erratic shifts made traditional gym routines impossible, so Samar focused on fitting extra activity into everyday life. He took the stairs instead of elevators, walked briskly during breaks, and did quick sets of squats and lunges at home. On his days off, he explored local hiking trails, combining exercise with the mental refreshment that comes from being in nature.

3. **Stress Management**

The hospitality industry often triggers high stress—managing staff schedules, dealing with customer complaints, and keeping track of inventory. Samar adopted simple mindfulness exercises before each shift. Pausing for a moment of deep breathing whenever he felt overwhelmed helped him avoid stress-related snacking and headaches.

4. **Sleep**

Rotating shifts threw Samar's internal clock off balance. His solution was to make sure his sleeping environment was dark, quiet, and free of electronic devices. He used earplugs and blackout curtains for daytime sleep and aimed for a minimum of 7 hours in each 24-hour cycle.

5. **Avoiding Harmful Substances**

Samar occasionally drank high-caffeine, high-sugar energy drinks. He replaced them with unsweetened iced tea and green tea. He also limited alcohol—common in hospitality culture—to once a week, opting for lower-sugar options when he did indulge.

6. Social **Bonds and Connections**

Samar joined an online community focused on weight loss and heart health. Sharing meal ideas, workout tips, and success stories inspired him and bolstered his motivation. Whenever he felt discouraged, supportive messages from fellow members reminded him he was not alone in his journey.

Outcome

Over the course of a year, Samar lost 40 pounds and brought his blood pressure back into a healthy range. His doctor applauded his progress and noted dramatic improvements in his cardiovascular risk factors. Feeling lighter both physically and mentally, Samar was ready to tackle the demands of the restaurant world with renewed confidence.

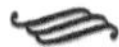

Conclusion

These 5 patients—Aarav, Shilpa, Nikhil, Ria, and Samar—offer a glimpse into how lifestyle medicine can transform heart health and reduce risk factors. Although each person's story is unique, the core elements of their success remain the same:

- **Diet:** Emphasise whole foods, limit sugar and sodium, and choose healthy fats.

- **Physical Activity:** Focus on consistent, enjoyable movement that fits your schedule.

- **Stress Management:** Explore practical coping strategies such as meditation, breathing exercises, journaling, or hobbies.

- **Sleep:** Prioritise steady, restful sleep to help the heart and body recover.

- **Avoiding Harmful Substances:** Reduce or eliminate tobacco, excessive alcohol, and stimulants.

- **Social Bonds and Connections:** Lean on the support of family, friends, colleagues, or online groups for motivation.

By weaving these 6 pillars into everyday life, profound healing and prevention become achievable. Lifestyle medicine does not just mask symptoms—it empowers people to actively nurture their own health, habit by habit.

Conclusion

Conclusion: A Heartfelt Path to Lifelong Wellness

As we reach the end of this transformative journey towards better heart health, it is important to remember that true wellness emerges from a harmonious blend of multiple factors. A holistic approach that weaves together balanced nutrition, regular exercise, effective stress management, restorative sleep, and meaningful social connections provides a solid foundation for maintaining a strong and vibrant heart. By nurturing each of these areas equally, we empower ourselves not only to protect our cardiovascular health but also to enhance our overall quality of life.

Embracing a Holistic Lifestyle

A vital lesson learned throughout this guide is that no single strategy can fully support heart health in isolation. Instead, genuine progress lies in combining various elements—like a nutrient-dense diet and consistent physical activity—into a comprehensive lifestyle. As highlighted earlier, "A combination of nutritious meals and regular physical activity lays the foundation for a heart-healthy lifestyle, empowering individuals to take control of their well-being." This synergy ensures that our efforts produce lasting, meaningful benefits for both body and mind.

Building Sustainable Habits

While taking the first step towards healthier living is commendable, sustaining those changes is just as crucial. Lasting improvement arises from turning intentions into daily practices that fit seamlessly into our routine. Even small modifications—such as choosing whole-grain bread over refined alternatives—can accumulate over time, leading to significant positive changes. As we have seen, "Small changes, like opting for whole-grain bread instead of refined options, can have a cumulative effect that significantly improves heart health over time." By focusing on these gradual shifts, we cultivate a lifestyle that supports our heart health effortlessly.

Fostering Supportive Relationships

Good heart health is influenced not only by what we do individually but also by our connections with others. Strong social ties provide invaluable emotional support and encouragement for maintaining a healthy lifestyle. Sharing workout goals with friends, celebrating milestones, or having someone to accompany us on a brisk walk can make the journey more enjoyable and keep us motivated. As previously mentioned, "Sharing fitness goals with friends not only bolsters motivation but also fosters a supportive environment that nurtures emotional resilience and heart health." In this way, our relationships become powerful catalysts for lasting, positive change.

Prioritising Mental and Emotional Well-Being

Emotional wellness and stress management are inseparable from physical health, particularly when it comes to the heart. Daily pressure, if left unaddressed, can undermine even the healthiest lifestyle choices. Incorporating mindfulness exercises, meditation, and simple relaxation techniques into our everyday routine can have a profound impact on reducing stress levels. As emphasised, "Engaging in mindfulness practices can drastically reduce stress levels, leading to a more vibrant emotional state that directly influences heart health." By proactively caring for our mental well-being, we lay a firm foundation for our cardiovascular system to thrive.

Looking Ahead

These core principles—integrating a holistic lifestyle, establishing sustainable habits, creating strong social bonds, and giving mental health its due attention—offer a clear and confident path forward. They remind us that safeguarding our hearts is not a fleeting task, but rather a lifelong commitment to health and happiness. May the insights shared here encourage you to take charge of your cardiovascular journey and pass this knowledge on to those around you, sparking a chain reaction of better health in your community.

About the Author

Dr. Jitesh Arora is a renowned physician and a passionate advocate for heart health. As the founder of a leading hospital in Rudrapur, Uttarakhand, he has dedicated his career to helping high-risk individuals reduce—and even reverse—serious cardiac conditions, not just through medication but with a holistic, lifestyle-centered approach.

A Holistic Approach to Heart Health

With years of hands-on clinical experience, Dr. Arora has developed a groundbreaking **Lifestyle Modification Program** that combines cutting-edge medical research with real-life success stories. His proven methodology integrates:

- **Smart Nutrition** – Practical, heart-friendly dietary changes

- **Stress Management** – Simple yet effective techniques for a balanced mind

- **Sustainable Exercise Habits** – Realistic movement strategies for lasting heart health

This holistic framework empowers individuals to take control of their well-being—one step at a time.

The Healthy Heart Blueprint: A Science-Backed Guide

In his transformative book, *The Healthy Heart Blueprint*, Dr. Arora distills his expertise into an easy-to-follow, science-driven guide. With a focus on education and prevention, he shares actionable strategies that help readers safeguard their heart health and reclaim their vitality.

A Trusted Voice

Dr. Arora's unwavering commitment to patient empowerment and evidence-based care has made him a trusted authority in the field. His work inspires individuals to take proactive steps toward a healthier, longer, and more vibrant life.

For personalized guidance, expert insights, or any heart-health-related questions, feel free to reach out to Dr. Jitesh Arora at **drjitesharora@gmail.com.**

Here's to a future filled with energy, resilience, and a healthy heart!

Appendix

Practical Tools, Resources, and Checklists

The following appendix is designed to help you put into action the heart health principles and strategies introduced in **The Healthy Heart Blueprint**. Whether you are looking for a quick-reference guide, daily trackers, or extra resources, these tools will support your ongoing journey toward a stronger, more resilient cardiovascular system.

A. Heart-Healthy Action Checklists

1. Daily Heart Care Checklist

- **Morning Routine:**
  - Drink a glass of water upon waking.
  - Spend 2–5 minutes doing gentle stretches or breathing exercises.
  - Eat a balanced breakfast (e.g., oatmeal with berries, whole-grain toast with avocado).

- **Midday Checkpoint:**
  - Fit in 10–15 minutes of physical activity (a quick walk, stair climbing, or desk exercises).
  - Choose a nutrient-dense lunch (including veggies, lean protein, and whole grains).
  - Check your posture – relax shoulders, align spine, and take a few deep breaths.

- **Afternoon Reset:**
  - Take a stress management break (e.g., mindfulness app, breathing exercise).
  - Hydrate with water or unsweetened tea instead of sugary drinks.
  - Opt for a healthy snack, such as nuts, fruit, or yogurt.

- **Evening Wind-Down:**

  - Spend at least 30 minutes on a heart-friendly activity: a brisk walk, easy yoga, or stretching.

  - Limit screen time and bright lights before bed.

  - Reflect on the day's wins and challenges in a simple journal.

- **Before Bed:**

  - Set a consistent bedtime to aim for 7–9 hours of sleep.

  - Practice a brief relaxation technique (progressive muscle relaxation, guided meditation).

  - Prepare for tomorrow (pack a healthy lunch, lay out workout clothes).

Use this checklist each day to stay focused on small, cumulative steps that nurture a healthy heart. Consistency in daily habits can yield remarkable long-term benefits.

2. Weekly Heart Health Planner

Day	Physical Activity	Meal Planning & Prep	Stress/Relaxation Activity	Social Connection
Mon				
Tue				
Wed				
Thu				
Fri				
Sat				
Sun				

- **How to Use This Table:**

  - **Physical Activity:** Schedule workouts or active breaks (e.g., gym sessions, walks, bike rides).

  - **Meal Planning & Prep:** Note which meals you will cook, batch cook on certain days, or meal prep tasks.

  - **Stress/Relaxation Activity:** Pencil in meditation, yoga, or simple breathing exercises.

- **Social Connection:** Plan family activities, calls with friends, or community events.

Filling this out weekly provides structure and accountability. It also helps you track and balance efforts across all areas of your heart health journey.

B. Heart-Healthy Grocery Essentials

1. **Produce (Fruits & Vegetables)**

   - **Leafy Greens:** Spinach, kale, collard greens
   - **Cruciferous Veggies:** Broccoli, cauliflower, Brussels sprouts
   - **Colourful Veggies:** Carrots, bell peppers, tomatoes, zucchini
   - **Berries:** Blueberries, strawberries, raspberries
   - **Citrus Fruits:** Oranges, grapefruits, lemons
   - **Others:** Apples, pears, bananas, avocados

2. **Whole Grains**

   - **Oats (rolled or steel-cut)**
   - **Brown Rice, Quinoa, Barley**
   - **Whole-grain bread or pasta**
   - **Millet, Buckwheat**

3. **Lean Proteins & Plant-Based Options**

   - **Poultry (skinless chicken or turkey)**
   - **Fish (salmon, mackerel, sardines, trout)**
   - **Legumes (lentils, beans, chickpeas)**
   - **Tofu, Tempeh**
   - **Low-fat or Greek yogurt**

4. **Healthy Fats**

   - Olive Oil, Avocado Oil
   - Nuts (almonds, walnuts, pistachios)

- Seeds (chia, flax, pumpkin, sunflower)

- Avocados

5. **Seasonings & Extras**

   - **Herbs & Spices:** Turmeric, cumin, basil, oregano, garlic, and ginger

   - **Low-sodium broths or stocks**

   - **Vinegars (balsamic, apple cider, red wine)**

   - **Lemon or lime juice for flavour**

Use this list to guide weekly shopping. Focusing on fresh, whole foods and limiting processed items helps maintain optimal heart health.

C. Portion Control Guidelines

- **Handy Visual Cues:**

  - **Protein (meat, poultry, fish):** About the size of your palm.

  - **Whole Grains or Starches:** About the size of a clenched fist.

  - **Fruits:** One piece of fruit or about a fistful of berries.

  - **Vegetables:** Aim for at least half of your plate at each meal.

  - **Healthy Fats:** About the size of your thumb (e.g., salad dressing, nut butter).

- **Practical Strategies:**

  - Use smaller plates and bowls to avoid over-serving.

  - Start meals with vegetables or a salad.

  - Eat slowly, pausing between bites to let satiety cues register.

  - Pack leftovers before you start eating (especially with large restaurant portions).

D. Quick Exercise Routines

1. **"10-Minute Office Circuit"**

   - **Chair Squats (1 minute):** Stand up from your chair and sit back down, repeating continuously.

   - **Desk Push-Ups (1 minute):** Place hands on the desk, step feet back, and perform push-ups at an incline.

   - **Wall Sit (30 seconds):** Slide your back down a wall and hold as though sitting on an invisible chair.

   - **Marching in Place (1 minute):** Lift knees high; swing arms to elevate heart rate.

   - **Calf Raises (1 minute):** Stand on your toes, then lower down; repeat.

   - **Repeat the circuit as time permits.**

2. **"At Home 15-Minute Routine"**

   - **Jumping Jacks or Marching (2 minutes):** Warm up your body and get your heart rate up.

   - **Bodyweight Squats (1 minute):** Keep your back straight and knees behind your toes.

   - **Lunges (1 minute):** Alternate legs, stepping forward or backward with control.

   - **Plank (30 seconds – 1 minute):** Keep your core tight, body straight from head to heels.

   - **Rest (30 seconds).**

   - **Push-Ups (1 minute):** On the floor or on your knees for modification.

   - **Side Plank (30 seconds each side):** Focus on engaging your core.

   - **Cool Down (2 minutes):** Gentle stretching for legs, arms, and back.

Adjust repetitions and durations to match your fitness level. Even brief bouts of activity boost cardiovascular health, especially when repeated consistently.

E. Stress Management and Relaxation Tips

1. **Breathing Exercises:**

    - **Box Breathing:** Inhale for 4 counts, hold for 4, exhale for 4, hold for 4. Repeat several times.

    - **Diaphragmatic Breathing:** Breathe in deeply through the nose, feeling your abdomen expand; exhale slowly through the mouth.

2. **Mindfulness or Meditation:**

    - Set aside 5–10 minutes to focus on your breath or use a guided meditation app (e.g., Headspace, Calm).

    - Try the "Body Scan" meditation to notice tension and release it progressively.

3. **Progressive Muscle Relaxation:**

    - Tense and relax each muscle group from your toes to your head, pausing to note the difference between tension and relaxation.

4. **Journaling:**

    - Spend a few minutes writing down worries, goals, or gratitudes. This helps process emotions and reduce mental clutter.

5. **Creative Outlets:**

    - Drawing, painting, playing an instrument, or listening to music can soothe the mind and lower stress hormones that impact the heart.

F. Recommended Apps & Online Resources

- **Nutrition & Meal Planning:**

    - **MyFitnessPal** (Calorie and nutrient tracking)

    - **Lose It!** (Food logging and weight management)

- **Exercise & Activity Tracking:**
  - **Fitbit, Garmin, Apple Health** (Wearable trackers with integrated apps)
  - **Nike Training Club** (Free guided workouts)
- **Stress Management & Mindfulness:**
  - **Calm, Headspace, Insight Timer** (Guided meditations and sleep support)
  - **Breathe2Relax** (Structured breathing exercises)
- **Sleep Tracking & Improvement:**
  - **Sleep Cycle** (Analyses sleep patterns, gentle wake up alarms)
  - **Pzizz** (Combines music, voice-overs, and sound effects for better sleep)
- **Heart Health Information & Community Support:**
  - **American Heart Association (AHA)**: www.heart.org
  - **Centers for Disease Control and Prevention (CDC) – Heart Disease**: www.cdc.gov/heartdisease

Use these digital tools to track progress, find motivation, and stay informed about heart health best practices.

G. Frequently Asked Questions (FAQs)

1. **How quickly can I expect to see changes in my heart health?**
   - Some benefits, like reduced blood pressure or improved blood sugar levels, can appear within a few weeks of consistent lifestyle changes. Others, such as significant weight loss or lowered cholesterol, may take a few months. Remember, every positive step adds up over time.

2. **Do I need to completely cut out all fats and carbs to protect my heart?**
   - Not at all. Focus on choosing **healthy fats** (e.g., olive oil, avocados, nuts) and **complex carbohydrates** (e.g., whole grains,

vegetables, legumes). Avoid trans fats, excessive saturated fats, and refined carbs to support better cholesterol levels and overall heart function.

3. **What if I don't have time for a full workout?**

   - Short, frequent activity bursts can be just as effective. Try breaking your exercise into 10–15-minute sessions throughout the day—walk during breaks, do quick bodyweight exercises at home, or take the stairs instead of the elevator.

4. **How can I cope with stress eating or emotional eating?**

   - Practice mindfulness around meals: pause before eating to check if you are truly hungry or just stressed. Keep healthy snacks on hand (fruit, nuts, yogurt) and address the root cause of stress through meditation, journaling, or counselling rather than reaching for food.

5. Is it okay to enjoy occasional treats or comfort foods?

   - Yes. An all-or-nothing approach often backfires. Aim for an 80/20 or 90/10 balance, where most of your choices are heart-healthy, allowing room for occasional indulgences without guilt.

6. **How do I maintain motivation for long-term lifestyle changes?**

   - Set realistic, specific goals (like walking 10,000 steps daily or cooking 4 healthy dinners per week). Track your progress with apps or journals. Celebrate small victories along the way and involve friends or family in your journey for added support and accountability.

H. References & Suggested Reading

- American College of Cardiology. (n.d.). **Guidelines for the Prevention of Cardiovascular Disease**.

- American Heart Association (n.d.). www.heart.org

- Dean Ornish, M.D. (2008). **The Spectrum: A Scientifically Proven Programme to Feel Better, Live Longer, Lose Weight, and Gain Health.**

- Esselstyn, C. B. Jr. (2007). **Prevent and Reverse Heart Disease: The Revolutionary, Scientifically Proven, Nutrition-Based Cure.**

- Pischke, C. R., Scherwitz, L., Weidner, G., & Ornish, D. (2008). "Long-term effects of lifestyle changes on well-being and cardiac variables among coronary heart disease patients." *Health Psychology*, *27*(5).

- World Health Organisation. (n.d.). **Cardiovascular Diseases (CVDs)**. www.who.int

These sources offer additional scientific insights and practical ideas to deepen your understanding of heart health.

Final Note on Sustaining Your Progress

An effective heart health strategy is not a one-time fix but a **lifelong journey**. This appendix gives you practical tools and frameworks to keep your momentum strong:

- **Use checklists** and planners to stay organised.

- **Maintain variety** in your exercise routines and meal choices.

- **Stay mindful** of portion sizes, emotional triggers, and the value of meaningful connections.

- **Celebrate each milestone**, no matter how small—every healthy meal, every walk, every meditation session strengthens your heart's resilience.

By merging knowledge with consistent action and supportive relationships, you will create a lifestyle that not only improves your cardiovascular health but also enriches your overall quality of life. Here is to a healthier, happier heart!

Glossary

Below is a concise glossary of key medical and cardiovascular terms mentioned throughout this book. Refer to these definitions whenever you need quick clarity.

1. **Metabolic Syndrome**

   A cluster of conditions—including high blood pressure, elevated blood sugar, excess body fat around the waist, and abnormal cholesterol or triglyceride levels—occur together, increasing the risk of heart disease, stroke, and type 2 diabetes.

2. **Atherosclerosis**

   A condition in which fatty deposits (plaques) build up on the inner walls of the arteries, narrowing them and restricting blood flow. Over time, this can lead to chest pain, a heart attack, or a stroke.

3. **Arrhythmias**

   Abnormal heart rhythms are caused by changes in the electrical impulses that control the heartbeat. These can range from harmless «skipped beats» to life-threatening irregularities like ventricular fibrillation.

4. **Endothelium**

   The thin layer of cells lining the interior surfaces of blood vessels. A healthy endothelium helps regulate blood pressure, blood clotting, and immune function, while an unhealthy one contributes to vascular disease.

5. **LDL (Low-Density Lipoprotein) Cholesterol**

   Often termed «bad» cholesterol. High levels of LDL contribute to plaque buildup in arteries, increasing the risk of heart attack and stroke.

6. **HDL (High-Density Lipoprotein) Cholesterol**

   Known as "good" cholesterol, it helps remove excess cholesterol from thebloodstream,transportingitbacktotheliverforprocessingorexcretion.

7. **Triglycerides**

   A type of fat (lipid) found in the bloodstream. Elevated levels often coincide with other conditions, such as obesity and metabolic syndrome, and can raise the risk of heart disease.

8. **Free Radicals**

   Unstable molecules are produced during normal metabolic processes or when exposed to certain environmental factors (e.g., pollution, tobacco smoke). Excessive free radicals can cause oxidative stress and damage cells and tissues.

9. **Omega-3 Fatty Acids**

   Essential fats are found in foods like fish (e.g., salmon, mackerel) and certain seeds (e.g., flax, chia). They help reduce inflammation, lower triglyceride levels, and support healthy blood vessel function.

10. **Inflammation**

    The body›s natural response to injury or infection. Chronic, low-grade inflammation can damage arteries and contribute to heart disease, among other chronic conditions.

11. **Hypertension (High Blood Pressure)**

    A persistent elevation of blood pressure in the arteries. Over time, uncontrolled high blood pressure can damage blood vessel walls and lead to serious cardiovascular issues.

12. **Insulin Resistance**

    A state in which the body›s cells become less responsive to insulin, a hormone regulating blood sugar. Often a precursor to type 2 diabetes, it also raises the risk of heart disease.

13. **Cortisol**

    A stress hormone released by the adrenal glands. While helpful in short bursts, persistently high cortisol levels can elevate heart rate and blood pressure and contribute to inflammation.

14. Antioxidants

Compounds that neutralise free radicals, helping to protect cells and tissues. Common antioxidant-rich foods include berries, leafy greens, and nuts.

15. Portion Control

Managing the amount of food eaten in a single sitting helps maintain a healthy weight and avoid excess calorie intake—both essential for supporting heart health.

16. Endorphins

Hormones produced in the brain that act as natural painkillers and mood elevators, often released during exercise, laughter, and other positive experiences.

17. Heart Rate Variability (HRV)

The variation in time between each heartbeat. A higher HRV indicates better cardiovascular fitness and an adaptive autonomic nervous system.

18. Sleep Apnoea

A sleep disorder characterised by pauses in breathing or shallow breathing during sleep. Untreated, it can lead to high blood pressure, arrhythmias, and other heart-related issues.

19. Mindfulness

The practice of staying present and fully engaged in the moment, often through techniques such as breath awareness or meditation, helps reduce stress and protect heart health.

20. Chronic Stress

A long-term form of stress resulting from ongoing pressures that seem unrelenting. Chronic stress can elevate blood pressure, increase inflammation, and damage blood vessels.

21. Statins

A class of medications used to lower LDL ("bad") cholesterol. While effective, they can reduce levels of CoQ10 in the body, sometimes necessitating supplementation.

22. Dietary Supplements

Products taken to add specific nutrients or compounds to the diet, such as omega-3 fatty acids, vitamins, minerals, or antioxidants. They are not replacements for a healthy lifestyle but can help fill nutritional gaps.

23. Coenzyme Q10 (CoQ10)

A naturally occurring antioxidant found in cells that is crucial for energy production, especially important for high-energy-demand organs like the heart.

24. Probiotics

Beneficial bacteria that support gut health. A balanced gut microbiome can positively affect overall health, including regulating inflammation that impacts the heart.

25. Familial Hypercholesterolaemia

A genetic disorder characterised by high LDL ("bad") cholesterol from birth. This significantly increases the risk of early heart disease and requires specialised care and sometimes genetic counselling.

Use this glossary to boost your understanding of important terms as you progress on your journey to a healthier heart. If you come across additional terminology or have further questions, consult a trusted medical professional or reputable health resources for clarification.

www.ingramcontent.com/pod-product-compliance
Lightning Source LLC
Chambersburg PA
CBHW021555150726
47990CB00006B/2553